Integrating Gerontological
Content Into Advanced
Practice Nursing Education

Carolyn Auerhahn, EdD, ANP, GNP-BC, FAANP, is a Clinical Associate Professor and Coordinator of the Geriatric and Adult Geriatric Nurse Practitioner Programs at New York University, College of Nursing. She also serves as the Associate Director and Director for Advanced Practice Initiatives at the Hartford Institute for Geriatric Nursing, also at NYU College of Nursing. Carolyn has been an ANP and a GNP for over 25 years. She has been actively engaged in the teaching of nurse practitioner students for more than 20 years and, prior to joining the faculty at NYU, held academic positions at Yale University School of Nursing and Columbia University School of Nursing. She received her Diploma in Nursing from the Bellevue School of Nursing in 1966, her BS (Nursing) from Pace University Lienhard School of Nursing in 1979, and her MS as an ANP from Columbia University School of Nursing in 1981. In 1996, she received an EdD in Health Education from Teachers College, also at Columbia University. In her clinical practice Carolyn has introduced the NP role in places where it was unknown and "paved the way" for other NPs, pioneered new and evolving aspects of the role, and brought national attention to the NP. She was inducted as a Fellow in the American Academy of Nurse Practitioners in 2006.

Carolyn is a Co-Project Investigator on the American Association of Colleges of Nursing/NYU Hartford Institute for Geriatric Nursing Advanced Practice Registered Nurse Initiative "Transitioning to Adult-Gerontology APRN Education: Ensuring the APRN Workforce is Prepared to Care for Older Adults." She is also a Co-Course Director for The Consortium of New York Geriatric Education Centers/Mount Sinai School of Medicine Brookdale/James J. Peters VA Medical Center GRECC: "Advanced Course in Geriatrics and Palliative Care for Frontline Primary Care Providers." She is one of the editors of the *Geriatric Nursing Review Syllabus: A Core Curriculum in Advanced Practice Geriatric Nursing*, Second Edition, published by the American Geriatrics Society. She has also published more than 30 peer-reviewed journal articles and seven book chapters. Carolyn has served as a consultant on several Health Resources and Services Administration grants for adult/gerontological NP programs. She has served as an international consultant regarding gerontological advanced practice nursing to schools of nursing in Japan, Korea, Taiwan, the Netherlands, Iceland, Brazil, and Colombia, in addition to more than six schools of nursing in the United States. She has been an active participant in the New York Academy of Medicine: Age-friendly New York City Initiative, chair of the National Organization of Nurse Practitioner Faculty's Geriatric SIG, chair of the Gerontological Advanced Practice Nurses Association's education committee, and a member of the American Nurses Credentialing Center: Gero-NP Task Force.

Laurie Kennedy-Malone, PhD, GNP-BC, FAANP, FAGHE, is a Professor and Director of the Adult/Gerontological Nurse Practitioner Program at The University of North Carolina at Greensboro. Laurie has been a certified gerontological nurse practitioner for over 25 years. She received her BSN in nursing and sociology from Worcester State College, Worcester, MA, in 1981 and her master's degree as a gerontological nurse practitioner from The University of Lowell in MA in 1982. She received her PhD in Nursing from The University of Texas in Austin in 1990. She has received numerous grants from the Health Resources and Services Administration for the nurse practitioner program at UNCG. She was one of the recipients of the John A. Hartford and American Association of Colleges of Nursing (AACN) Geriatric Nursing Education Project: Enhancing Gerontological/Geriatric Nursing for Advanced Practice Nursing Program.

She is one of the authors of *Management Guidelines for Nurse Practitioners Working with Older Adults* published by F.A. Davis. She is a Fellow of the Association of Gerontology in Higher Education and the American Academy of Nurse Practitioners. Laurie served on the National Expert Panel that developed the *Nurse Practitioner and Clinical Nurse Specialist Competencies for Older Adult Care* and the Advisory Committee for the AACN's Creating Careers in Geriatric Advanced Practice Nursing. She currently serves on the AACN/NYU Hartford Institute APRN Initiative "Transitioning to Adult-Gerontology APRN Education Ensuring the APRN Workforce Is Prepared to Care for Older Adults." She received the AACN and the John A. Hartford Foundation Institute 2007 Awards for Excellence in Gerontological Nursing Education: Geriatric Nursing Faculty Champion and the 2006 National Conference of Gerontological Nurse Practitioner's Excellence in Education Award.

Integrating Gerontological Content Into Advanced Practice Nursing Education

CAROLYN AUERHAHN, EdD, ANP, GNP-BC, FAANP
LAURIE KENNEDY-MALONE, PhD, GNP-BC, FAANP, FAGHE

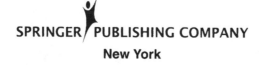

SPRINGER PUBLISHING COMPANY
New York

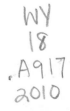

Springer Publishing Company, LLC
11 West 42nd Street
New York, NY 10036
www.springerpub.com

Acquisitions Editor: Margaret Zuccarini
Senior Editor: Rose Mary Piscitelli
Cover design: Steven Pisano
Composition: Sweety Singh, Aptara

ISBN: 978-0-8261-0536-3

E-book ISBN: 978-0-8261-0537-0

10 11 12 13/ 5 4 3 2 1

CIP data is on file at the Library of Congress

Printed in the United States of America by Hamilton Printing

I dedicate this book to my husband Brett Auerhahn for always being there, to my parents Mildred and Albert Szymanski who always faced the challenges of aging "head-on," to my older patients who taught me so much, and to the older adults of today and tomorrow for whom this book has ultimately been written.

Carolyn Auerhahn

I would like to dedicate this book to my husband Chris and son Brendan for their support and encouragement during this endeavor. To my parents Nancy and Edward Kennedy, who are models of successful aging.

Laurie Kennedy-Malone

Contents

Contributors

Caroline Dorsen, MSN, FNP-BC
Clinical Instructor
Coordinator, Adult Primary Care Master's and Post Master's Programs
New York University College of Nursing
New York, New York

Evelyn G. Duffy, DNP, G/ANP-BC, FAANP
Assistant Professor
Director of the Adult-Gerontological Nurse Practitioner Program
Associate Director of the University Center on Aging and Health
Frances Payne Bolton School of Nursing, Case Western Reserve University
Cleveland, Ohio

Marilyn J. Hammer, PhD, DC, RN
Assistant Professor
New York University College of Nursing
New York, New York

Kathleen Meyer, DNP, GCNS, BC
Instructor, Master of Science in Nursing Program
Frances Payne Bolton School of Nursing, Case Western Reserve University
Cleveland, Ohio

Leslie-Faith Morritt Taub, DNSc, ANP-C, GNP-BC, CDE, CBSM
Assistant Professor
Division of Graduate Studies
University of Medicine and Dentistry of New Jersey, School of Nursing
Newark, New Jersey

M. Catherine Wollman, MSN, GNP-BC
Coordinator, Adult and Geriatric Nurse Practitioner Program
Neumann University, Division of Nursing and Health Sciences
Aston, Pennsylvania

Foreword

The aging of the U.S. population is a reality that presents multiple challenges to this nation, not the least of which is the need to have a highly educated workforce of health professionals able to deliver high-quality and appropriate care to the population of older adults. Advanced practice registered nurses (APRNs) are an essential part of the workforce to deliver care to our nation's older adults. Given the important role APRNs have, and will continue to play, in providing high-quality care to older adults, the advanced practice community has developed radically transformative recommendations about the education of any APRN who will care for adults.

The results of the APRN Consensus Process mandate that any APRN educated to care for adults must have an extensive exposure to the unique practice requirements of caring for older adults. The reality is that almost all practice today is practice with an older adult population. Additionally, given the widespread recognition that the expertise for care of geriatric patients cannot reside only in the armamentarium of geriatric specialty-prepared clinicians, a national process has begun to transform the education of APRNs who will now be prepared as adult/gerontology APRNs in roles as nurse practitioners or clinical nurse specialists.

This timely book provides a unique resource for our nation's advanced practice nursing clinicians, students, and educators and is representative of the lifelong commitment to care of older adults embodied in the work of its authors, Dr. Carolyn Auerhahn and Dr. Laurie Kennedy-Malone. I am pleased and honored to be able to write this foreword to share with the readers of this important work my respect for Carolyn and Laurie. I also am pleased to offer my endorsement for its importance to our profession and the goals of the APRN community to ensure that all clinicians caring for adults have a high level of knowledge and the skills for care of older adults.

I had the privilege of meeting Carolyn through our mutual work in our respective organizations to address concerns about how we will better prepare nurses in advanced practice to care for older adults. Her zeal and commitment to this work were a valuable asset to us at the American Association of Colleges of Nursing (AACN) as we sought to educate faculty about the needs of older adults. AACN's strong commitment to development of faculty for their roles as knowledge-based educators of professional nurses who will provide high-quality, safe, and appropriate care to older adults is shared by Carolyn. Her work to develop case studies for graduate students evolved to collaboration with the AACN in development of the competencies for adult/gerontology practice. Moreover, her commitment to this important work has continued as she has collaborated with us in the development of resources and tools that will provide faculty in the APRN programs with the capacity to teach this important content. What started with a mutually shared commitment to the best care of this population, however, has evolved to a respect for her work, her commitment, her expertise, and her energy in this important effort.

Dr. Kennedy-Malone's life's work has been devoted to education, practice, and research in care of older adults. She is nationally and internationally recognized for her expertise in gerontology and is highly sought after as a consultant by APRN faculty. The quality of her work has also been recognized by her induction as a Fellow of the Association of Gerontology in Higher Education. Laurie has been an integral part of a number of AACN initiatives focused on faculty development and APRN education in care of older adults, and in 2007 she received the AACN and John A. Hartford Foundation Institute Award for Excellence in Gerontological Nursing Education: Geriatric Nursing Faculty Champion. A major focus of Laurie's collaboration with AACN has been the development of APRN competencies for care of older adults and this continues with the development of competencies for adult/gerontology practice and resources for APRN faculty.

The Institute of Medicine (IOM) report, *Retooling for an Aging America,* issued a challenge to all health professionals, not just APRNs, to prepare our new clinicians for the reality of a changing demographic. Dr. Auerhahn and Dr. Kennedy-Malone have taken up this challenge and developed multiple resources to ensure that APRNs are engaged fully and competently in this new care reality. The IOM report predicts that the current 12% of the U.S. population over the age of 65 will increase to 20% in the near future. Chronic illness and high use of health care services are common in this population and, despite this reality, older adults often receive care that is disconnected, complex, and uncoordinated. APRNs are essential to overcoming these challenges. As our nation's nurse educators respond to this reality, they will be challenged to reframe and dramatically revise and improve the content and learning experiences that frame the journey to advanced practice. This text will provide an important source of support for ensuring that APRN educators can address this need.

I am delighted that the development of this important text coincides with the growing efforts among the APRN community of providers to transform how we are prepared for practice and how we focus on the needs of a significant component of the patient population. This text is a natural adjunct that will assist faculty and students to achieve the goal of being well prepared for care of older adults. Carolyn Auerhahn and Laurie Kennedy-Malone are to be commended for this leading-edge work to ensure that nurses in general, and APRNs specifically, have the requisite knowledge, skills, and commitment to care for older adults.

Geraldine Polly Bednash, PhD, RN, FAAN
Chief Executive Officer/Executive Director
American Association of Colleges of Nursing

Preface

We are on the brink of a major health care crisis. As the Baby Boomers transition into old age, we will see a doubling or tripling, by the year 2030, in the number of adults over the age of 65. This unprecedented increase alone would qualify as a crisis, but when it occurs within the context of an "across-the-board" shortage of health care providers with the necessary knowledge and skills to provide care for this growing population, the magnitude of this crisis exceeds that of any we have seen in modern times. The Institute of Medicine (2008) in its recent report, *Retooling for an Aging America: Building the Health Care Workforce*, calls for fundamental reform in the training of health care providers and an increase in the production of providers qualified to care for older adults in order to address this workforce shortage. Advanced practice nurses (APNs) have always taken a proactive approach in response to crises and difficult challenges and we are doing that now.

The intended audience for this text is faculty in all nongerontological advanced practice nursing (APN) programs. It is a *must-have* resource given the projected changes in population demographics (aging of the Baby Boomers), proposed changes in the regulation of APNs, and potential changes in accreditation of APN programs. The audience includes not only adult and family APNs but also acute care, women's health, psychiatric mental health, holistic, palliative, pediatrics, and other specialties. Graduates of all these programs have the potential for caring for older adults, whether directly as a patient or indirectly as a family member or caregiver. Therefore, gerontological content must be included in the curricula of these programs as well.

However, there are many questions that must be answered and resources to answer those questions may not seem to be readily available. What are the priorities? What content requires the most emphasis? How do you engage students in an area in which you yourself have little engagement? This text offers the answers to these questions and more.

This text will facilitate the integration of much needed content about care of older adults into their curricula by faculty in nongerontological APN programs. It provides clear "user-friendly" guidelines *written by APN faculty for APN faculty*. It focuses on ways to incorporate the content into already existing programs without requiring major curricular changes. The authors are sharing almost 50 years of combined experience of struggling with the answers to these and other curricular questions as well as specific examples of strategies for inclusion of gerontological content.

The text is divided into three sections. Section I: Key Factors Related to Integration of Gerontological Content Into Advanced Practice Nursing Curriculum presents content related to the rationale/need to do this, challenges to inclusion of this content, strategies to address these challenges, and gerontological content that needs to be included. Section II: Resources for Integration of Gerontological Content Into Advanced Practice Nursing Curriculum provides detailed lists of print media and internet resources. Section III: Methodology for Integration of Gerontological Content Into Advanced Practice Nursing Curriculum includes a discussion of a competency-based framework and process for the integration of gerontological content. In addition, there are three chapters that focus on course-specific gerontological content, competencies addressed by this content, teaching/learning strategies, and evaluation methods for integration of this content into graduate nursing core, APN core, and specialty courses. Strategies to facilitate the inclusion of clinical experiences focused on care of older adults are included as well. This section also includes examples, written by other APN faculty, of successful integration of this content into several nongerontological APN programs.

Adding content to an already burgeoning APN curriculum can be challenging given the numerous retraints we have on our time and resources. The authors have addressed many of the challenges and offered overall general strategies for curricular enhancement of gerontological content needed for APNs managing the care of older adults. By integrating content across the graduate program using blended technology and the multiple gerontological resources recommended in this text, faculty can begin to ensure that students gain gerontological competency.

Carolyn Auerhahn, EdD, ANP, GNP-BC, FAANP
Laurie Kennedy-Malone, PhD, GNP-BC, FAANP, FAGHE

Acknowledgments

I thank my colleagues at the Hartford Institute for Geriatric Nursing, Mathy Mezey, Malvina Kluger, and Ethel Mitty for their encouragement and support, and my students who over the years have always kept me on target.

Carolyn Auerhahn, EdD, ANP, GNP-BC, FAANP

I would like to acknowledge the assistance of Margaret Markham and Susan Roberts in reviewing part of this manuscript.

Laurie Kennedy-Malone, PhD, GNP-BC, FAANP, FAGHE

Integrating Gerontological Content Into Advanced Practice Nursing Education

SECTION I

Key Factors Related to Integration of Gerontological Content Into Advanced Practice Nursing Curriculum

CHAPTER 1

The Aging of America and Its Impact on Advanced Practice Nursing Education

Carolyn Auerhahn

One of the major health care challenges of the 21st century will be the provision of quality, comprehensive, cost-effective care for a rapidly increasing number of older adults. The elderly population in the US is expected to double, if not triple, by 2030 with the greatest growth in those 80 years of age and older. The prevalence of chronic illness and disability, especially in those over the age of 85, is expected to skyrocket. Health care costs are expected to escalate at a rate not seen before (Administration on Aging [AoA], 2008).

Despite the recent increased emphasis on gerontology in medical and nursing curricula, the emergence of specialized care units in hospitals, and the development of alternative long-term care options, the demand will still overwhelm the supply of qualified providers (Institute of Medicine [IOM], 2008). That leaves us with the burning question: Who will care for this ever-growing number of older adults? It is obvious that in order to address this challenge, more health care providers with the knowledge and skills to provide care for this growing population are needed.

This chapter will provide an overview of these issues. Recommendations from a recent Institute of Medicine (IOM) report will be discussed. The role of advanced practice nurses (APN) in addressing this challenge and the proposed new model for the regulation of APNs, including its mandate to include more gerontology in all APN programs, will also be discussed. Finally, the purpose of the text and an overview of its contents will be presented.

OVERVIEW OF THE ISSUES

Changes in Population Demographics

By now the statement "the Boomers are aging" has become commonplace in our society. But who exactly are the Boomers? Between 1946 and 1964 there was a dramatic increase in births that was dubbed the "Baby Boom," and the term "Boomer" was coined to describe those born during this time period. Driving many public services, such as schools and health care, the Boomers have dominated U.S. culture since the end of World War II.

The first wave of the Boomers became eligible for Social Security in January 2008 and will turn 65 in 2011. Life expectancy for someone turning 65 in 2009 is, on average, an additional 19.0 years (AOA, 2008), and given past trends it is a reasonable expectation that this number will increase as we go forward. The aging of the Boomers will result in an extraordinary increase in the population over 65, predicted to be a doubling or tripling of the older population by 2030 (AOA, 2008).

Not only will the number of older adults increase, there will also be an increase in the prevalence of chronic illness. Sixty percent of the aging Boomers will be managing more than one chronic condition. Obesity will be a major problem affecting more than one out of every three Boomers. It is projected that one in four will have diabetes and one in two will have arthritis (American Hospital Association [AHA], 2008).

In addition, the Boomers are different from earlier generations in several ways that will impact health care delivery. They are more racially and ethnically diverse than previous generations. Approximately 20% are members of minority groups, and this percentage is expected to increase as the immigrant population continues to expand and the disparity in projected life span between minorities and non-Hispanic Whites continues to decrease. Boomers are more educated and, in general, more active participants in their health care. They also have higher expectations of service and will demand more innovative, personalized health care programs (AHA, 2008). These differences will mandate health care delivery systems and will expect a workforce with knowledge and sensitivity to cultural differences and their impact on health care, and will require a philosophy that is patient-focused, flexible, and individualized.

Health Care Workforce

The demands on the U.S. health care system by those over the age of 65 will be greater than they have ever been before (AHA, 2008). In a recent report, *Retooling for an Aging America: Building the Health Care Workforce,* the IOM (2008) issued the urgent warning that the U.S. health care system is ill-prepared to meet these demands. The projected shortage of a health care workforce capable of delivering quality care to the growing number of older adults is a major area of concern. Providing care for the older adult is not merely providing care for an adult who is older. It requires specialized knowledge and skills, as well as a proactive attitude and approach.

The projected workforce shortage applies to all health care disciplines. In medicine, there is an estimated need for 36,000 board-certified geriatricians by 2030. As of 2007, there were only 7,128 board-certified geriatricians, which was a 22% decrease since 2000. Current enrollments in geriatric fellowship programs do not indicate that this decline will be eliminated in the near future. One estimate predicts that if current trends in growth and attrition continue, there will only be approximately 7,750 board-certified geriatricians by 2030. A similar shortage is also predicted for geriatric psychiatry (IOM, 2008).

The situation for advanced practice nursing is comparable to that of medicine. There is already a shortage of gerontological APNs relative to the current number of older adults, and recent trends in the preparation of APNs do not look promising for the future. Although a 60% decline in the number of gerontological nurse practitioner (NP) graduates from 2002 to 2004 stabilized by 2007, the numbers are still insufficient to meet the current, let alone the growing, need. Due to the low numbers of gerontological clinical nurse specialist (CNS) graduates, no statistical trends have been noted. The current shortage of gerontological APNs is probably a direct result of a national trend to prepare APNs with a broader scope of practice, such as family NPs or adult health CNSs (Thornlow, Auerhahn, & Stanley, 2006).

The shortage of health care professionals prepared to care for older adults is not limited to medicine and advanced practice nursing. Less than 1% of registered nurses, pharmacists, and physician assistants specialize in geriatrics. Social work reports that only 4% of social workers specialize in geriatrics (IOM, 2008).

IOM RECOMMENDATIONS

In its report *Retooling for an Aging America: Building the Health Care Workforce,* the IOM (2008) presents recommendations to address the imminent shortage in the health care professional workforce. The three major points of this report are: the training and use of the workforce needs to undergo fundamental reform; the workforce needs to be large enough and must possess the necessary skills to care for the growing population of older adults; and this workforce shortage needs to be addressed quickly and efficiently. A key recommendation is the expansion of the definition of the health care workforce to include not only health care professionals and direct-care workers, but also informal caregivers and patients.

IOM's recommended approach consists of three parts. First, knowledge and skills of the newly defined workforce in care of older adults need to be ensured. There also needs to be an increase in efforts focused on the recruitment and retention of health care professionals and caregivers who are specialists in the care of older adults. Last, and certainly not least, plans for improvement in health care delivery to older adults need to be developed. Suggested strategies include the requirement of basic competence in the care of older adults for licensure or certification of health care workers, and the inclusion of common geriatric conditions, such as decreased mobility and impaired vision and hearing, in all workforce training programs. The report also strongly recommends the use of nursing homes, patients' homes, or assisted living facilities as training sites for medical students and resident physicians (IOM, 2008).

As discussed previously, our health care system is facing new challenges related to population differences, challenges that are greater than ever before—a workforce shortage and a workforce that is ill-prepared to meet these demands. The IOM recommendations offer guidelines that will be useful to all health care professions as we work together to address the health care challenges of the 21st century.

ROLE OF ADVANCED PRACTICE NURSING

We are faced not only with the burgeoning growth of our population aged 65 and over, but with a population that will require caregivers to be knowledgeable about and sensitive to cultural differences, to be patient focused, and to be flexible in their approach to care. These are characteristics that are integral to APN roles and require only that we continue to practice as we always have and to educate our future generations to do likewise.

The workforce deficits are, however, another matter. As the data show, it is unrealistic to expect only APNs who have graduated from gerontological APN programs to care for older adults (Thornlow, Auerhahn, & Stanley,

2006). APNs have always taken a proactive approach in response to difficult challenges and we are doing that again now. Creative strategies have already been employed and initiatives have been begun by APNs to address this critical issue.

One strategy recently instituted to address this issue in the short term is the recent change in eligibility requirements for the American Nurses Credentialing Center's (ANCC) Gerontological NP Certification Exam. Alternative eligibility criteria, which include education and practice requirements, have been developed by ANCC that allow nationally certified adult, acute care, and family NPs to apply for a second certification as an ANCC Gerontological NP (ANCC, 2009). This strategy will increase the numbers of NPs currently in practice who have achieved national recognition for their expertise in delivering quality care to older adults. It may also encourage other practicing NPs who already care for older adults to acquire the additional knowledge and skills necessary to achieve that recognition.

Another strategy, which could prove to be the long-term answer to the workforce issue for APNs, is to include a foundation in gerontology in the education of all APNs who provide care to older adults (Thornlow et al., 2006). A first step in the implementation of this strategy was taken in 2004 by the American Association of Colleges of Nursing (AACN) with the publication of the *Nurse Practitioner and Clinical Nurse Specialist Competencies for Older Adult Care.* With funding from the John A. Hartford Foundation, a set of gerontological competencies was developed for both NPs and CNSs in specialties that provide care to older adults but who are not specialists in gerontology. The intent of this document is to outline the competencies and critical content that should be included in nongerontological APN educational programs in order to prepare their graduates to safely and competently care for older adults (AACN, 2004). This document will be discussed in detail in Chapter 6 of this text.

This strategy has also been evident in recent efforts focused on proposed changes in the regulation of APNs. A new model for regulation of APNs has been developed by the Advanced Practice Nursing Consensus Work Group (Consensus Group) and the National Council of State Boards of Nursing APRN Committee (NCSBN). Work on this project by these two bodies has been ongoing for several years. Initially begun independently of one another, representatives of the Consensus Group and NCSBN joined forces to form what is called the APRN Joint Dialogue Group (Joint Dialogue Group). The product of the Joint Dialogue Group, "Consensus Model for APRN Regulation: Licensure, Accreditation, Certification & Education"

(Consensus Document), was reached by consensus, and unanimous agreement was obtained on most of the recommendations in the document. It defines APN practice and describes the APN regulatory model, including the titles to be used. It also defines specialty and population foci. Strategies for implementation of the new model are also presented (APRN & NCSBN, 2008). An overview of the new model and a discussion of the Joint Dialogue Group's recommendations as they relate to this text are presented in the following. The full document is available on the AACN Web site and can be accessed at www.aacn.nche.edu/.

NEW MODEL FOR REGULATION OF ADVANCED PRACTICE NURSING

In the new model presented in the Consensus Document, regulation has been defined to include licensure, accreditation, certification, and education, which is commonly known as LACE. The ultimate goal of LACE is to protect the public and promote patient safety. The recommendations in the Consensus Document address issues that APNs are dealing with currently, but they also focus on the future. The strength of this new model is that it was developed through the collaboration of APN certifying agencies, accrediting organizations, public regulators, educators, and employers. The goal of the Consensus Document is that it will provide guidance for informed decision making by all parties when confronted with current and future APN issues (APRN & NCSBN, 2008).

The new model, as shown in Figure 1.1, has three levels. The first level consists of the four APN roles that currently exist: certified registered nurse anesthetist (CRNA), certified nurse-midwife (CNM), clinical nurse specialist (CNS), and certified nurse practitioner (CNP). In the new model, the four roles will all have the same title of advanced practice registered nurse (APRN). The second level consists of six populations: family/individual across the life span, adult-gerontology, neonatal, pediatrics, women's health/gender-related, and psychiatric/mental health. Education, certification, and licensure will bring together the APRN core and role competencies within the context of at least one of the six populations. Licensure will be as independent practitioners in the role and population for which they have been educated and certified (Figure 1.2). The third level consists of APN specialties such as oncology, palliative care, and orthopedics. Specialties will serve to expand or deepen practice within the APRN's

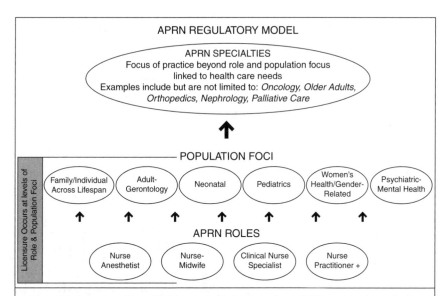

Figure 1.1. APRN Regulatory Model.

Source: APRN Consensus Work Group and National Council of State Boards of Nursing APRN Advisory Committee (APRN and NCSBN). (2008). Consensus Model for APRN Regulation: Licensure, Accreditation, Certification & Education.

specific population. They will not be a basis for licensure. Curriculum for the specialties will be developed by the nursing profession and assessment of competence in the specialties will be the responsibility of professional certifying organizations, not state boards of nursing (see Figure 1.2) (APRN & NCSBN, 2008).

Several of the Joint Dialogue Group's recommendations are especially relevant to the purpose and content of this text. The first of these is the designation of one of the populations as adult-gerontology. This population is defined as being inclusive of the young adult to the older adult, with specific mention made of the frail elderly (APRN & NCSBN, 2008). The recommendations also state that "APRNs educated and certified in the

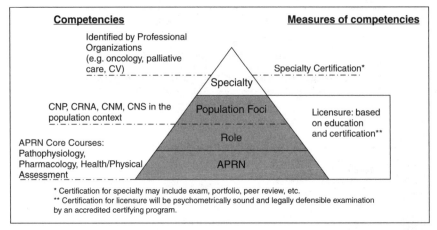

Figure 1.2. Relationship among educational competencies, licensure, and certification in the role/population foci and education and credentialing in a specialty.
Source: APRN Consensus Work Group and National Council of State Boards of Nursing APRN Advisory Committee (APRN and NCSBN). (2008). Consensus Model for APRN Regulation: Licensure, Accreditation, Certification & Education.

adult-gerontology population are educated and certified across both areas of practice" (APRN & NCSBN, 2008, p. 9).

While older adults are currently within the scope of practice for adult NPs and adult health CNSs, gerontological content in these educational programs is not consistent and often lacks fundamental content necessary to care for older adults, especially for the most frail in this group. The numbers of adult NP and adult health CNS educational programs are significantly greater than those that prepare gerontological APNs (Thornlow et al., 2006). By requiring all adult NP and adult health CNS educational programs to provide essentially the same gerontological content as current gerontological NP and CNS programs, the number of APNs capable of providing safe, comprehensive care to older adults would increase exponentially.

In addition, the Joint Dialogue Group recommends that "all APRNs in any of the four roles providing care to the adult population, e.g., family or gender specific, must be prepared to meet the growing needs of the older adult population" and "the education program should include didactic and clinical education experiences necessary to prepare APRNs with these enhanced skills and knowledge" (APRN & NCSBN, 2008, p. 9). While this recommendation does not specifically require the same amount or depth of gerontological content as in the adult-gerontology population focus, it does provide for the inclusion or augmentation of gerontological content in these programs. This would result in an additional component of the APN workforce that is better equipped to address the health care challenges associated with the growing population of older adults.

Recommendations regarding the process and requirements for APN program accreditation are also included in the Consensus Document. Although they are essentially the same as current requirements, they are clearly defined within the context of the new model of APRN role and population.

The new model for regulation of advanced practice nursing is an important initiative that would enhance our ability to successfully meet the challenges of the health care professional workforce shortage head on. It addresses the three major points of the IOM (2008) report: the training and use of the workforce needs to undergo fundamental reform; the workforce needs to be large enough and possess the necessary skills to care for the growing population of older adults; and this workforce shortage needs to be addressed quickly and efficiently. It is also consistent with the IOM's suggested strategy that basic competence in care of older adults be a requirement for licensure or certification of all health care workers (IOM, 2008).

The new model is targeted for full implementation in 2015. The Joint Dialogue Group continues to meet to discuss the formation of a permanent LACE structure that will provide guidance for implementation. In order for full implementation to occur, however, the individual state boards of nursing, schools of nursing, certifying organizations, and accrediting bodies will need to evaluate what changes need to be made and what specific actions will be necessary to bring about these changes (Stanley, 2009).

PURPOSE AND OVERVIEW OF THE TEXT

As APN faculty, we are facing a number of significant challenges in APN education that need to be addressed over the next several years. The expected changes in population demographics will result in a shortage of health care providers qualified to care for the older adult population. We are responsible for the production of future APNs and, consequently, will need to find ways to increase the number of graduates qualified to care for this population. The proposed change in the regulation of advanced practice nursing, specifically the requirement of more gerontological content in all

APN programs, is one way to accomplish this. However, this presents another challenge to faculty in nongerontological APN programs: the unique nature of older adults.

As mentioned earlier, providing care for the older adult is not merely providing care for an adult who is older. It requires specialized knowledge and skills, as well as a proactive attitude and approach. Understanding the importance of not treating aging changes as a disease and not attributing disease to older age is a critical skill for all APNs. For example, geriatric syndromes, while a familiar concept to APN faculty with gerontological specialization, are often foreign concepts to nongerontological APN faculty. Depression, dementia, delirium, sleep disturbances, constipation, incontinence of bladder and bowel, polypharmacy, and decreased vitality are examples of syndromes that may not be addressed in nongerontological curricula. In addition, in the older adult, common diseases present in uncommon ways and diseases that are rare in younger adults may be the diagnosis in the older adult.

The purpose of this text is to facilitate the integration of gerontological content into curricula by faculty in nongerontological APN programs. It provides clear "user-friendly" guidelines and detailed lists of resources. In addition, it focuses on ways to incorporate the content into already existing programs without requiring major curricular changes.

The content of the text is divided into three sections. Section I discusses key factors related to the integration of gerontological content into advanced practice nursing curriculum, such as the preceding discussion of the rationale/need for this, challenges to the inclusion of this content, strategies to address these challenges, and the gerontological content that needs to be included. Section II consists of annotated lists of both print media and Internet resources. Section III presents a competency-based framework for the integration of gerontological content, and specific guidelines for integration of this content into graduate nursing and APN core courses, as well as specialty courses within the context of this framework. Also included in Section III are exemplars or "success stories" from nongerontological APN programs that have been successful in integrating gerontological content.

REFERENCES

Administration on Aging, U.S. Dept. of Health and Human Services (AOA). (2008). *A profile of older Americans: 2008*. Retrieved May 23, 2009, from http://www.aoa.gov/AoARoot/Aging_Statistics/Profile/index.aspx

American Association of Colleges of Nursing (AACN). (2004). *Nurse practitioner and clinical nurse specialist competencies for older adult care.* Washington, DC: Author.

American Hospital Association (AHA). (2008). *When I'm 64: How Boomers will change healthcare.* Retrieved May 23, 2009, from www.aha.org/aha/content/2007/pdf/070508-boomerreport.pdf

American Nurses Credentialing Center (ANCC). (2009). *Gerontological nurse practitioner application alternative criteria.* Retrieved August 2, 2009, from http://www.nursecredentialing.org/Documents/Certification/Application/NursingSpecialty/GerontologicalNursePractitionerAlternativeCritiera.aspx

APRN Consensus Work Group and National Council of State Boards of Nursing APRN Advisory Committee (APRN & NCSBN). (2008). *Consensus model for APRN regulation: Licensure, accreditation, certification and education.* Retrieved May 23, 2009, from www.aacn.nche.edu

Institute of Medicine (IOM). (2008). *Retooling for an aging America: Building the health care workforce.* Washington, DC: The National Academies Press. Retrieved May 23, 2009, from www.nap.edu

Stanley, J. (2009). Reaching consensus on a regulatory model: What does this mean for APRNs? *Journal for Nurse Practitioners, 5*(2), 99–104.

Thornlow, D. K., Auerhahn, C., & Stanley, J. (2006). A necessity not a luxury: Preparing advanced practice nurses to care for older adults. *Journal of Professional Nursing, 22,* 116–122.

CHAPTER 2

Challenges to Inclusion of Gerontological Content and Strategies to Address These Challenges

Carolyn Auerhahn

Laurie Kennedy-Malone

Evelyn G. Duffy

The responsibility of providing care to older adults is included in the scope of practice of all APNs who provide care to adults, regardless of specialty or setting. Inherent in the pervasive problem of the growing shortage of APNs with the necessary knowledge and skills to provide safe, effective care to older adults has been the less-than-adequate quantity and quality of gerontological content in many nongerontological APN programs, the graduates of which will be expected to provide care for older adults. The end result is that the APN expertise necessary to provide care for the growing complex health care needs of the diverse aging population has been hampered by compromised curricula and by limited clinical exposure to older adults across the continuum of care.

In this chapter, challenges, and often barriers, to preparing competent APNs with the necessary gerontological knowledge, skills, and attitudes are presented. While not unique to nursing education, the challenges identified here are often the result of the lack of a faculty champion, in this case, one who recognizes the need for inclusion of specialized content and clinical experiences for students caring for older adults in nongerontological APN programs. This chapter will also delineate strategies for overall curricular revision directed at integrating gerontological content into the APN curriculum. Recognizing that curricular enhancement is time consuming and requires "buy in" from faculty and administration, recommendations are presented to ease the frustration often encountered when changes in nursing curriculum are mandated. Finally, the need to identify early on those stakeholders who will support the curricular change is suggested as a means of garnering support beyond the nursing faculty.

CHALLENGES

It has been our experience that there are a number of challenges APN faculty encounters when attempting to include more gerontological content in nongerontological APN courses and program curricula. Those most commonly identified by APN faculty are the addition of more content within established credit limits, lack of interest in this content by students and faculty, faculty-knowledge deficit regarding gerontological content, lack of a clear understanding by faculty of the unique nature of the older adult, and faculty discomfort with their own knowledge base. These challenges are consistent with those found across health care professions (Cummings & Galambos, 2002; Gilje, Lacey, & Moore, 2007; Plowfield, Raymond, & Hayes, 2006; Rosen, Zlotnik, & Singer, 2003; Rosenfeld, Bottrell, Fulmer, & Mezey, 1999; Ryan & McCauley, 2004/2005; Wesley, 2005). Other challenges identified in a study of gerontological education in social work, which may also have relevance to nursing, include lack of organizational commitment to effect curricular-wide change, lack of substantive faculty incentives for effecting curricular change, and competing organizational and faculty special interests (Rosen et al., 2003).

Additional Content

Adding more content within established credit limits is a very real concern voiced repeatedly whenever this is suggested. Faculty state they find it difficult to include, within their current credit load, all that they *already* must include. The reality is that an increase in the number of credits translates directly into increased tuition costs, which, in turn, impacts recruitment and retention of students.

Interest in Content

The lack of interest in gerontological content by students and faculty is another challenge that is frequently cited by faculty. We have faced this challenge as well when teaching this content to nongerontological APN students. All too often gerontology is only seen as caring for the frailest of elders in long-term care institutions. This point of view diminishes the rich diversity offered by older adults and belies their presence in almost every health care setting. There is considerable evidence in the literature that health care providers may exhibit attitudes, beliefs, and behaviors that are associated with agism against older patients (Cummings & Galambos, 2002; Latimer & Thornlow, 2006; Nelson, 2005; Ryan & McCauley, 2004/2005; Thornlow, Latimer, Kingsborough, & Arietti, 2006; Wesley, 2005).

In the broad sense, agism can be defined as "prejudice by one age group toward other age groups" (Butler, 1969, p. 243). It is a subjective experience and can apply to members of all age groups, such as a teenager's distrust of anyone over the age of 30 or vice versa. When applied to older adults, it may be manifested as "distaste for growing old, disease, disability; and fear of powerlessness, 'uselessness,' and death" (Butler, 1969, p. 243).

Ageist attitudes and beliefs are not limited to health care providers. We live in a culture that values youth. Most Americans hold ageist attitudes and beliefs and are reluctant to accept aging gracefully for themselves. Messages related to this unease with aging may be so well learned that people respond to them on the subconscious level (Butler, 1969; Kite & Wagner, 2004; Nelson, 2005). In health care settings this may impact significantly on decision making regarding care and services that an older patient receives.

Because this challenge may be reflective of deeply held beliefs, attitudes, and/or values about older adults, it can be more difficult to address than some of the other challenges. Creative problem solving and strategies focused on beliefs, attitudes, and values will need to be utilized. Educational strategies focused on attitude change have been successful in undergraduate programs (Blais et al., 2006; Burbank et al., 2006)

Faculty Knowledge Base

Of the approximately 240,000 APNs in the United States (140,000 NPs and 73,000 CNSs) (Health Resources and Services Administration [HRSA], 2006), only 4,400 are certified in gerontological nursing (3,700 NPs and 668 CNSs) (American Nurses Credentialing Center [ANCC], 2006). While not representative of all APNs or all APN faculty, these statistics are useful in providing a general indication of formal APN preparation in gerontology. Without a basic foundation in gerontological content, faculty may have no reference point on which to build the development of this content in their programs.

Faculty may believe that aging is adequately covered in current nongerontological APN programs, citing "diagnosis and treatment of chronic illness" as evidence of this. While it is true that older adults suffer from multiple chronic illnesses, management of chronic illness is not equivalent to the essential gerontological content needed to provide safe, comprehensive care to older adults (Newell, Raji, Lieberman, & Beach, 2004). Without an understanding of this gerontological content, even good evidence-based care of chronic illness in an older adult can result in less than optimal outcomes. Adding content on dementia, palliative care, or polypharmacy may increase the knowledge of the management of problems common to older adults, but only including select topics misses the crucial elements of basic gerontological considerations.

Understanding the Unique Nature of the Older Adult

A major challenge to the integration of gerontological content occurs when faculty do not understand the unique nature of the older adult: their prevalence in all settings of care; the variation among them; and their unique biological, psychological, and social needs that require a different approach to care. Older adults are not just adults who are older. While all 3-year-olds are expected to reach certain milestones at predicted times, older adults do not reflect predictable patterns of development (Duthie, 2007). There is greater variation among older adults at the same chronological age. For older adults, functional health, not chronological age, is an important measure of age (Touhy, 2008). For example, some 80-year-olds are climbing mountains, while others are not even capable of feeding themselves.

Physiologically there are declines that come with aging that are unique to each individual. In fact, even within a single individual, organ systems age at different rates (Landefeld et al., 2004). Psychologically, older adults are the product of a lifetime of coping with their life stages. Life's rewards as well as its losses and disappointments result in each older adult becoming "uniquely themselves" (Touhy, 2008, p. 598). Social needs are altered by retirement, relocation, and the disease or death that affects the older adult or those close to them. The combination of biological, psychological, and social challenges to the aging adult strongly impacts their care. In order to teach students to provide optimal care to older adults, faculty need a clear understanding of their unique nature.

Faculty Discomfort With Their Knowledge Base

The discomfort that comes with integrating new content into a course or curriculum is not exclusive to nursing. The concept of faculty discomfort served as the theoretical model for a study of teachers required to implement curricular reform in mathematics (Fryckholm, 2003; Miller Mlcak, 2009). It was hypothesized that discomfort may develop with the teacher's changing role and the resulting vulnerability when content is relatively new. As a result of the investigation, Fryckholm (2003) identified four domains: cognitive discomfort, belief-driven discomfort, pedagogical discomfort, and emotional discomfort. Two of these domains are especially relevant to the focus of this text. One domain, cognitive discomfort, is faculty discomfort as a result of uncertainty with content. Another domain, emotional discomfort, results from faculty's vulnerability due to a new curriculum being implemented. While a similar study of these concepts has not included nursing faculty, anecdotal evidence indicates that it applies to APN faculty as well. Feedback we have received from some faculty indicates a significant degree of apprehension regarding the complexities of older adults. Given the challenge brought forth by the new regulatory model requiring the integration of gerontology in all APN programs, it is likely that most nongerontological APN faculty will understandably face a certain degree of discomfort.

STRATEGIES TO FACILITATE CURRICULAR REVISION

As APN educators, we are now faced with the task of enhancing the curriculum to address the needs of our rapidly growing, diverse aging population. Given that we are often required to add content to our curriculum reflecting the changes in health care and the cliental we serve, it is challenging, even daunting at times, to increase content in our individual programs to meet the requirements of accrediting bodies and/or national organizations. The blueprint for the strategies that we offer in this chapter can be used when faculty needs to increase additional content areas that must be strengthened in the future. The deliberate inclusion of gerontological content in the graduate nursing core courses, the APN core requirement of advanced health/physical assessment, advanced physiology and pathophysiology, and

Exhibit 2.1. Strategies to Enhance Infusion of Gerontological
Nursing Curricula

- Require readings that pertain to gerontological nursing.
- Designate a percentage of test questions to reflect the inclusion of gerontological nursing.
- Provide students with Web-based resources and community linkages.
- Encourage students with an interest in gerontology to focus written assignments on gerontological nursing issues.
- Require a designated amount of clinical time to be devoted to caring for older adults in all clinical settings.
- Measure competence in the care of older adults in didactic and clinical courses.

Source: Kennedy-Malone, L., Penrod, J., Kohlenberg, E., Letvak, S., Crane, P., Tesh, A., Kolanowski, A., Hupcey, J., & Milone-Nuzzo, P. (2006). Integrating gerontology competencies into graduate nursing programs. *Journal of Professional Nursing, 22*(2), p. 124. Reprinted with permission of the publisher, Elsevier Inc.

advanced pharmacology, and the specialty courses can be achieved for all APN students using the overall strategies listed in Exhibit 2.1.

Two other identified challenges to the integration of gerontological content into nongerontological APN programs are faculty knowledge deficit and faculty discomfort with the knowledge base. The most useful strategy to address these challenges is faculty development (Latimer & Thornlow, 2006). Faculty development workshops that deliver state-of-the-art, gerontological, evidence-based content are necessary to enable nongerontological APN faculty to integrate this content into their courses (Green, Dezendorf, Lyman, & Lyman, 2005; Kennedy-Malone et al., 2006; Thornlow, Latimer, Kingsborough, & Arietti, 2006). Ideally, these workshops should be taught by an expert interdisciplinary panel of faculty from gerontological nursing, geriatric medicine and pharmacy, geriatric social work, and other geriatric specialties (Thornlow et al., 2006). Once the knowledge deficit is corrected, the faculty's discomfort with their knowledge base should improve as well.

Student lack of interest and agist attitudes toward older adults are difficult challenges to address. An initial strategy is to assess the students' preconceptions about aging and caring for older adults (Thornlow et al., 2006). Because APN students are registered nurses who practice predominately in acute care settings, their clinical experience with older adults has been with sick, debilitated patients and, as a result, their preconceptions of older adults may be mostly negative. Increased gerontological content alone can improve students' attitudes (Newell et al., 2004). Another strategy to counteract negative preconceptions is to present the gerontological content beginning with healthy older adults both in didactic courses and clinical practica (Thornlow et al., 2006), and progress to the frailest, most vulnerable older adults.

PROMOTING AND SUSTAINING GERONTOLOGICAL CURRICULAR INNOVATIONS

A key to success for integrating gerontological content across the nongerontological APN curriculum is to have an APN faculty champion. This is an APN faculty member who is not only familiar with the gerontological concepts that need to be embedded into the curriculum, but also the faculty who will obtain the "buy in" from others of the nursing faculty and in administration to offer continued support to sustain this important initiative. The faculty champion will need to become familiar with the strategies needed to integrate gerontological content into the APN curriculum, identify the resources that he/she is able to access at the university and in the community, and cultivate a working relationship with the other APN faculty that demonstrates his/her ability to lead the curricular change and the formative and summative evaluation process.

Also essential to the process of integrating gerontology into the nongerontological APN curriculum is gaining the assistance of a wide range of stakeholders that include students, alumni, potential and known employers, university gerontology colleagues, and community partners with a special interest in older adults. Additionally, seeking assistance from regional and national experts in gerontology and gerontological nursing is advantageous to the APN program that seeks to be on the forefront of modeling curricular innovations in integrating gerontology into the APN curriculum (Kennedy-Malone et al., 2006).

The notion of curricular review is not a new concept to APN faculty. Given the numerous challenges addressed earlier in this chapter, it is important to review strategies that can aid faculty directly with planning the revision. Exhibit 2.2 presents suggestions for faculty to consider before undertaking this process.

Exhibit 2.2. Strategies for Implementing Curricular Revisions
_____

- Curriculum revision always takes longer than you expect: Strategically plan timing.
- The "ideal" curriculum is easier to write than a "feasible" curriculum: Carefully evaluate resources and capacity.
- Faculty input is critical: Collect, incorporate, and acknowledge it.
- Usually, you cannot fix everything at once: Plan for incremental change.
- Plan adequate, but time-limited, discussion sessions: Keep focused.
- Summarize concerns at each meeting and, later, articulate how voiced concerns were addressed: Problematic issues will not go away.
- Engage the broadest faculty group involved in the change in the process: Do not create an "us versus them" situation.
- Acknowledge that some issues are entwined in programmatic decisions, but not resolved solely through curriculum revisions: Remember the bigger picture.
- Consider a wide range of stakeholders (including students, potential and known employers, in-house and external colleagues): Build coalitions to sustain your innovations.
_____

Source: Kennedy-Malone, L., Penrod, J., Kohlenberg, E., Letvak, S., Crane, P., Tesh, A., Kolanowski, A., Hupcey, J., & Milone-Nuzzo, P. (2006). Integrating gerontology competencies into graduate nursing programs. *Journal of Professional Nursing, 22*(2), p. 127. Reprinted with permission of the publisher, Elsevier Inc.

SUMMARY

The pervasive lack of gerontological APNs needed to care for our rapidly growing aging population has been documented for many years (Futrell & Mellio, 2005; Thornlow, Auerhahn, & Stanley, 2006) and despite numerous funded projects to prepare more gerontological APNs (Kennedy-Malone et al., 2006; Thornlow et al., 2006), it is clear now that the directive has moved away from simply ensuring that there is an adequate number of specialized gerontological APNs available to *requiring* that all APNs caring for older adults be competent to care for their special health care needs (Institute of Medicine [IOM], 2008; Stanley, 2009).

As the educators of the APNs of tomorrow, nursing faculty must overcome the challenges that may have prevented the growth of the geriatric nurse specialist in the past. We must embrace the change that is being mandated to us and begin to initiate the strategies recommended in this chapter to integrate gerontology competencies into APN programs (Kennedy-Malone et al, 2006). The framework for developing a competency-based gerontological integrated APN curriculum is presented in Chapter 6. Specific curricular strategies and resources for the graduate nursing core, APN core, and specialty courses are delineated in Chapters 7, 8, and 9.

Ultimately, older adults will benefit when all APNs managing the care of older adults matriculate through a program that has integrated gerontological content across the curriculum. "Their acquired competency in the care of older adults will enable them to deliver care relevant and safe in the workplace" (Kohlenberg, Kennedy-Malone, Crane, & Letvak, 2007, p. 43). The need for gerontological health care specialists remains (IOM, 2008), however, the proposed solution – to prepare gerontological competent APNs – is a reality that nursing faculty *can* achieve.

REFERENCES

American Nurses Credentialing Center (ANCC). (2006). *Annual report 2005: Building and sharing knowledge*. Silver Spring, MD: Author.

Blais, K., Mikolaj, E., Jedlicka, D., Strayer, J., & Stanek, S. (2006). Innovative strategies for incorporating gerontology into BSN curricula. *Journal of Professional Nursing, 22*(2), 98–102.

Burbank, P. M., Dowling-Castronovo, A., Crowther, M. R., & Capezuti, E. A. (2006). Improving knowledge and attitudes toward older adults through innovative educational strategies. *Journal of Professional Nursing, 22*(2), 91–97.

Butler, R. N. (1969). Age-ism: Another form of bigotry. *The Gerontologist, 9,* 243–246.

Cummings, S. M., & Galambos, C. (2002). Predictors of graduate social work students' interest in aging-related work. *Journal of Gerontological Social Work, 39,* 77–94.

Duthie, E. H., Katz, P. R., & Malone, M. L. (2007) *Practice of geriatrics* (4th ed.). Philadelphia: Saunders.

Futrell, M., & Mellio, K. D. (2005). Gerontological nurse practitioners: Implications for the future. *Journal of Gerontological Nursing, 31*(4), 19–24.

Fryckholm, J. (2003). Teachers' tolerance for discomfort: Implications for curricular reform in mathematics. *Journal of Curriculum and Supervision, 19*(2), 125–150.

Gilje, F., Lacey, L., & Moore, C. L. (2007). Gerontology and geriatric issues and trends in U.S. nursing programs: A national survey. *Journal of Professional Nursing, 23*(1), 21–29

Green, R. K., Dezendorf, P. K., Lyman, S. B., & Lyman, S. R. (2005). Infusing gerontological content into curricula: Effective change strategies. *Educational Gerontology, 31*(2), 103–121.

Health Resources and Services Administration (HRSA). (2006). *The registered nurse population: Findings from the March 2004 national sample survey of registered nurses.* Washington, DC: Department of Health and Human Services.

Institute Of Medicine (IOM). (2008). *Retooling for an Aging America: Building the health care workforce.* Washington, DC: The National Academies Press. Retrieved from www.nap.edu

Kite, M. E., & Wagner, L. S. (2004). Attitudes toward older adults. In T. D. Nelson (Ed.), *Ageism: Stereotyping and prejudice against older persons* (pp. 129–162). Cambridge, MA: MIT Press.

Kennedy-Malone, L., Penrod, J., Kohlenberg, E., Letvak, S., Crane, P., Tesh, A., Kolanowski, A., Hupcey, J., & Milone-Nuzzo, P. (2006). Integrating gerontology competencies into graduate nursing programs. *Journal of Professional Nursing, 22*(2), 122–128.

Kohlenberg, E., Kennedy-Malone, L., Crane, P., & Letvak, S. (2007). Infusing gerontological nursing content into advanced practice nursing education. *Nursing Outlook, 55*(1), 38–43.

Landefeld, C. S., Palmer, R. M., Johnson, M. A., Johnston, C. B., & Lyons, W. L. (Eds.). (2004). *Current geriatric diagnosis and treatment.* New York: McGraw-Hill.

Latimer, D. G., & Thornlow, D. K. (2006). Incorporating geriatrics into baccalaureate nursing curricula: Laying the groundwork with faculty development. *Journal of Professional Nursing, 22*(2), 79–83.

Miller Mlcak, E. A. (2009). Necessary discomfort. *Field Notes, 4*(3). Retrieved from http://www.bard.edu/mat/field-notes/archive.shtml?aid=885&pid=72

Nelson, T. D. (2005). Ageism: Prejudice against our feared future self. *Journal of Social Issues, 61*(2), 207–221.

Newell, D. A., Raji, M., Lieberman, S., & Beach, R. E. (2004). Integrating geriatric content into a medical school curriculum: Description of a successful model. *Gerontology and Geriatrics Education, 25*(2), 15–32.

Plowfield, L. A., Raymond, J. E., & Hayes, E. R. (2006). An educational framework to support gerontological nursing education at the baccalaureate level. *Journal of Professional Nursing, 22*, 103–106.

Rosen, A. L., Zlotnik, J. L., & Singer, T. (2003). The need to "gerontologize" social work education. *Journal of Gerontological Social Work, 39*(1), 25–36.

Rosenfeld, P., Bottrell, M., Fulmer, T., & Mezey, M. (1999) Gerontological nursing content in baccalaureate nursing programs: Findings from a national survey. *Journal of Professional Nursing, 15*(2), 84–94.

Ryan, M., & McCauley, D. (2004/2005). We built it and they did not come: Knowledge and attitudes of baccalaureate nursing students toward the elderly. *Journal of the New York State Nurses Association, 35*, 5–9.

Stanley, J. (2009). Reaching consensus on a regulatory model: What does this mean for APRNs? *Journal for Nurse Practitioners, 5*(2), 99–104.

Thornlow, D. K., Auerhahn, C., & Stanley, J. (2006). A necessity not a luxury: Preparing advanced practice nurses to care for older adults. *Journal of Professional Nursing, 22*(2), 116–122.

Thornlow, D., Latimer, D., Kingsborough, J., & Arietti, L. (2006). *Caring for an aging America: A guide for nursing faculty.* Washington, DC: American Association of Colleges of Nursing / John A. Hartford Foundation.

Touhy, T. A. (2008) Emotional health in late life. In P. Ebersole, P. Hess, T. A. Touhy, K. Jett, & A. S. Luggen (Eds.), *Toward healthy aging: Human needs & nursing response* (7th ed., pp. 597–638). St. Louis, MO: Mosby.

Wesley, S. C. (2005) Enticing students to careers in gerontology: Faculty and student perspectives. *Gerontology and Geriatrics Education, 25*, 13–29.

CHAPTER 3

Gerontological Content That Needs to Be Included

Carolyn Auerhahn

Laurie Kennedy-Malone

Evelyn G. Duffy

In order to provide safe, effective care to older adults, graduates of APN programs need to possess a knowledge base that is appropriate for care of older adults. It is the responsibility of faculty in APN programs to ensure that this occurs. However, as discussed in Chapter 2, there are several challenges to the integration of gerontological content into APN programs. The challenges that have the most relevance to the subject of this chapter are those related to faculty knowledge base and the unique nature of older adults. In order to be successful in integrating gerontological content in their courses, APN faculty must have a clear understanding not only of what needs to be included, but why it does. This chapter will discuss the content areas relevant to the older adult that must be included in APN programs and the rationale for doing so.

Although in recent years there have been several articles related to the integration of gerontological content into APN programs (Kennedy-Malone et al., 2006; Kohlenberg, Kennedy-Malone, Crane, & Letvak, 2007; Thornlow, Auerhahn, & Stanley, 2006), the evidence base related to specific gerontological content that needs to be included in APN courses is sorely lacking. An extensive search revealed only one study that expressly addressed this topic (Towner, 2006). In addition, although there are substantially more articles related to integration of gerontological content into nursing baccalaureate programs, there were no articles found that specifically addressed what content should be included. There have been some publications in the medical (AGS, 2002, 2004; Newell, Raji, Lieberman, &

Beach, 2004) and social work (Rosen, Zlotnik, Curl, & Green, 2000) literature addressing specific gerontological content that needs to be included in those programs. The content presented in this chapter will be based on the findings of the APN study, literature addressing medical school and social work curricula, and the expertise of the authors.

In the study conducted by Dr. Elizabeth M. Towner (2006) over a 3-year time period, the gerontological knowledge base of students entering an APN program was assessed based on knowledge and skills necessary for the baccalaureate-prepared nurse to provide safe, effective care to older adults. The results indicated that knowledge deficits related to gerontological content existed in the following areas: demographics; health policy; health care system services for the elderly; myths of aging; health promotion and risk factors; assessment of functional status; normal changes of aging versus pathological changes; geriatric syndromes; and advance directives (Towner, 2006). While this assessment was conducted essentially to evaluate gerontological content in baccalaureate nursing education, it has obvious implications for APN education. APN education and practice builds on the foundation of baccalaureate nursing education and practice. Therefore, the knowledge base necessary for APN graduates to deliver safe, effective care to older adults includes not only those aspects specific to APN practice such as diagnosis and management of illness, but also the content necessary for the baccalaureate-prepared nurse to deliver safe, effective care. If that knowledge is lacking, it must be included in APN programs whose graduates will care for older adults.

The areas of gerontological content specified in the medical and social work literature mirror many of the areas assessed in Towner's study. In two similar but separate publications, the American Geriatrics Society (AGS) issued geriatric curriculum guidelines for medical and osteopathic schools (AGS, 2002) and internal medicine residency programs (AGS Education Committee, 2004). Gerontological content areas included in these documents are: demographics and epidemiology; health policy and health care financing; health promotion; theories of aging; normal aging versus pathological changes; comprehensive geriatric assessment; geriatric syndromes and conditions; atypical presentation of illness; pharmacological changes related to aging; psychosocial issues; ethical issues; cultural aspects of aging; advance directives; and end-of-life care. The required gerontological content specified in the article by Newell, Raji, Lieberman, and Beach (2004) coincided with that of the AGS documents. Despite the fact that the scope of practice for social work varies from that of nursing and medicine, there are similarities in the gerontological content that is required in their graduate and undergraduate programs. In addition to content on psychosocial aspects of aging, culture and diversity, legal and ethical issues, health policy, and health care systems and resources, required content also includes normal changes of aging, theories of aging, health promotion concepts, and pharmacology in aging (Rosen et al., 2000).

This chapter will be divided into the following sections: economic, political, and social issues; legal and ethical issues; theories of physical aging; normal physical changes of aging; psychosocial needs; health promotion; diagnosis and management of episodic, acute, and chronic illness; atypical presentation of illness; and geriatric syndromes. Each section will describe the gerontological content and the rationale for its inclusion in APN programs.

ECONOMIC, POLITICAL, AND SOCIAL ISSUES

The key topics of gerontological content related to economic, political, and social issues that must be included in APN courses are: demography and epidemiology of aging, including the growth and heterogeneity of the older adult population; the mechanisms and implications of health care policies and financing for older adults; myths and stereotypes related to older adults and their impact on health care delivery; and cultural aspects of aging.

Demography and Epidemiology of Aging

By now it is common knowledge that the population over the age of 65 is growing rapidly. The main points related to this growth include the following. Between 1997 and 2007 the size of the older adult population increased by 11.2%. During that same time period, the number of people who will turn 65 over the next 20 years increased by 38%. Today one in every eight people in the United States is over the age of 65 and that number is expected to double or triple by 2030. Life expectancy is increasing and the greatest percentage in growth will occur in the population over the age of 85. The numbers of older ethnic and racial minorities will also increase. Older women outnumber older men and that trend is expected to continue. Approximately 30% of older adults living in noninstitutional settings, including half of the women over the age of 75, live alone. Although only about 4% of older adults live in institutional settings such as nursing homes, this number increases with age. More than 450,000 grandparents are primary caregivers for their grandchildren who share their homes (Administration on Aging [AOA], 2008).

Not only is the older adult population growing exponentially, the composition of the group is changing in several ways. As we go forward, we will see a blending of two very different cohorts of older adults. The older adults of today are often referred to as "survivors" because they have survived the Great Depression, several major wars, discrimination, poverty, and communicable diseases. They were the first to witness medical milestones such as the large-scale development of antibiotics and the enactment of legislation for civil rights, Social Security, Medicare, and Medicaid. In 2011, a new cohort of older adults will emerge—the earliest of the Baby Boomer generation will turn 65. This cohort is often referred to as "aging." They have a longer life expectancy and the major causes of death, many of which are preventable, have changed. They are also more racially and ethnically diverse and more educated than previous generations (AOA, 2008). Having lived with Social Security, Medicare, Medicaid, and medical advances as givens, and with economic matters better than the cohort before them, they have come to expect more from the health care system. These two cohorts will coexist for years to come resulting in a diverse group with different personalities, values, functional levels, expectations, and health care needs. As such, it is imperative that APN students learn about and understand current and projected demographic characteristics of this changing population in order to deliver safe, effective, and individualized care.

Health Care Policies and Financing for Older Adults

Older adults are living longer than ever before and the number of adults that continue to work past the age of 55 continues to increase. Social Security comprises 90% or more of income for about one-third of Social Security beneficiaries. More than 50% of older adults report more than one source of income, such as personal assets, private pensions, government employee pensions, and earnings. However, almost 10% of older adults are below the poverty level and there have been statistically significant increases in the number at or below the poverty level in recent years (AOA, 2008).

When questioned about their health status, approximately 70% of older adults report that it is good or better. Despite the increased risk for chronic disease in this population, the rate of functional decline has decreased in recent years. A decrease in the rates of nursing home residence has also been noted. This decrease may be due to improvements in health and functioning of older adults, other forms of residential care and services, and greater use of resources that help older adults remain in their homes. However, older adults continue to use more health care services than any other age group. Health care costs have risen significantly in recent years with drug costs alone doubling. Drug costs account for the largest percentage of out-of-pocket health care spending. The amount spent on out-of-pocket health care expenses has been shown to have an impact on access to care, health status, and quality of life (Federal Interagency Forum, 2008).

Almost all noninstitutionalized adults over the age of 65 are insured through Medicare. However, Medicare only covers about 50% of their health care costs, primarily the costs for acute care and physician services. The costs for prescriptions, dental care, and nursing homes come either from out-of-pocket or other payers. More than 50% of noninstitutionalized older adults have private health insurance and about 10% are also covered by Medicaid. Slightly more than half of Medicare beneficiaries in nursing homes also have coverage from Medicaid (AOA, 2008; Federal Interagency Forum, 2008). Although Medicare D, which was added in 2006, provides some prescription coverage, it still carries a monthly premium, co-pays, and a high deductible also known as the "donut hole."

APNs provide care to older adults in a number of health care settings. APNs whose scope of practice is as a primary care provider can be reimbursed directly for their services. Medicare will reimburse the APN primary care provider at a rate of 85% of the physician rate. Other insurers have varying policies regarding APNs. In order to provide safe, affordable care it is imperative that APNs, regardless of setting or scope of practice, have a clear understanding of health care policies and financing related to older adults. They need to know what is covered by Medicare and what is not. They also need to know what other coverage options are available in addition to Medicare so that they can educate and counsel their patients. Within this context, content about health care policies and financing related to older adults needs to be included in APN educational programs that prepare graduates to provide care to older adults. In addition, this is also important for graduates of all APN programs as these issues may indirectly impact their chosen population as well.

Myths and Stereotypes Related to Older Adults

There is considerable evidence that most Americans, including health care providers, have agist attitudes and beliefs against older adults (Cummings & Galambos, 2002; Kite & Wagner, 2004; Nelson, 2005; Ryan & McCauley,

2004/2005; Wesley, 2005). Various myths and stereotypes exist that may compromise care of the older adult. Examples of some common myths and stereotypes are presented in Table 3.1.

In health care settings agist attitudes and beliefs may impact significantly on decision making regarding care and services that an older patient receives. Therefore, it is important to address this issue in APN programs. The various myths and stereotypes related to older adults need to be identified, discussed especially with regard to their impact on patient care, and most importantly, refuted.

Cultural Aspects of Aging

As the older adult population becomes more culturally and ethnically diverse, it is increasingly important that health care providers become more attuned to different cultural characteristics and their impact on health care (Auerhahn, Capezuti, Flaherty, & Resnick, 2007). Areas of content that need to be included in APN programs include the influence of culture and ethnicity on the aging process, perceptions of health and disease, and access to health care. Emphasis needs to be placed on the demographics of ethnic older adults in the United States, risk factors and disease prevalence in these populations, and principles for providing culturally competent health care (AGS, 2002). It is also important to emphasize that within each culture there exist wide individual variations in beliefs, traditions, customs, and preferences in order to prevent stereotyping an older adult based on cultural or ethnic group (Auerhahn et al., 2007). In addition, of interest are the findings of wide variations in patterns of disease that remain largely unexplained in older adults from different cultural and ethnic groups and that persist in their descendents (World Health Organization [WHO], 1999).

LEGAL AND ETHICAL ISSUES

Health care in the United States is based on the principles of respect for autonomy, nonmaleficence, beneficence, and justice. However, their application varies among and within our subcultures, including that of older adults. For example, it is not uncommon for health care providers to defer decisions to an older adult's children even when the patient is cognitively intact and capable of making a decision. In addition, agist attitudes and

TABLE 3.1. Myths and Stereotypes Related to Older Adults

Myth/Stereotype	Fact
Older adults are all the same	Older adults are not all alike. They are a heterogeneous population with variations in biological, psychological, and social needs that require different approaches to care. There may also be significant variations among older adults of the same chronological age. For example, some 80-year-olds are climbing mountains, while others are not even capable of feeding themselves.
Old age is "ill age"	The majority of older adults are driven to live longer, healthier lives and remain physically fit well into old age. Preventive and health promotion measures can increase their ability to function independently into their 80s and 90s.
Mental ability declines with age	Cognitive decline is not a normal change of aging. Attitude, motivation, and health are key factors in cognition. Decreased cognitive ability found in some older adults is usually associated with multiple causes such as physiological imbalances, depression, inadequate social support, and environmental factors. Also, much of what is attributed to decreased intelligence is a loss of investment in life as well as the loss of significant others (Auerhahn, Capezuti, Flaherty, & Resnick, 2007).
Productivity declines with age	Productivity is related to a complex interaction of different factors including biological, psychosocial, and environmental factors. However, productivity is frequently equated with participation in the paid workforce. There is also an assumption that the decrease in numbers of older adults in paid positions is related to a decline in functional capacity, when it may actually be due to disadvantages in education, and training, and agism rather than to old age (WHO, 1999). In the United States, the retirement age is increasing and older adults are continuing to hold paying jobs well into their 70s and 80s. In addition, many older adults begin a second career after retirement, which is frequently as an unpaid volunteer.
Old age is sexless	Sexuality is an important part of life for both men and women throughout the adult life span. Sexual function is mediated by biological, psychological, and social factors and there are changes associated with aging. While these changes are a major source of anxiety for some older adults, with adequate education and counseling, they can continue to have an enjoyable sex life well into old age (Morley, 2006).

beliefs about the health of older adults may result in the denial of beneficial treatment to healthy older adults (Auerhahn et al., 2007).

Within this context there are several legal and ethical issues related to older adults that must be included in all APN educational programs. Compliance with HIPPA when caring for older adults needs to be reinforced. Permission still needs to be given by either the older patient or a designated health care proxy before talking to the family about the patient. A clear explanation of exactly what is and is not included in a power of attorney is also necessary. In addition to content about the various types of advance directives and DNR (do not resuscitate) orders, APN students need to know what is allowed under their states' laws. Including content related to the basic principles of health care ethics and older adults is essential, but teaching content about ethical issues is not always straightforward. The definition of what is ethical is shaped by numerous factors, such as cultural values and perspectives, religious beliefs and specific situations, and is highly individual. Topics such as euthanasia, assisted suicide, and health care rationing are examples of topics that tend to result in "lively" class discussions. However, these discussions afford an excellent teaching opportunity on the subject of ethics.

THEORIES OF PHYSICAL AGING

Why we age is a question that has yet to be answered definitively. There are numerous diverse theories of physical aging, including biochemical/molecular, cellular, and genetic, that attempt to answer this question (AGS, 2002). One widely accepted theory of physical aging is oxidative stress. According to this theory, the oxidation that occurs during the metabolic processes of the body results in the production of several chemicals called free radicals. Free radicals act as mediators for the accumulation of protein, lipid, and DNA damage to the cells over time. Other theories being investigated include age-acquired chromosomal alterations that lead to the expression of disease-related genes, immunologic causes such as deficits in T-cell function that predispose older adults to infections, a neuroendocrinological process similar to that related to the cortisol surge leading to death in spawning salmon, and developmental genetics causes, such as a genetically programmed induction of aging and activation of the aging gene (Auerhahn et al., 2007).

Another theory, first put forward by Dr. Robert M. Perlman in 1958, is called "The Aging Syndrome." This theory equates aging to a disease complex, the etiology of which is from internal and external environmental stressors. Assaults from these stressors result in pathological effects that are multiphasic and asymptomatic in the early stages. These effects build up over time causing cellular damage leading to partial or complete failure of target resistance. The final result of this process is the destruction of basic functional and/or structural organization (Perlman, 2003).

Knowledge about theories of physical aging is important because it contributes to the scientific basis of care of older adults. In addition, because age-dependent changes in cellular and organ functions vary from person to person with large interindividual variations (Auerhahn et al., 2007), it directly impacts patient care. Understanding the theoretical basis for the normal physical changes of aging will help the practicing APN to put presenting symptoms and clinical findings into the context of normal changes of aging versus pathological processes.

NORMAL PHYSICAL CHANGES OF AGING

Although there is no definitive answer to the question of why we age, there are definitive answers related to what happens as we age. There are well-defined physical changes that occur due to normal aging. These changes happen as a result of the following mechanisms: the biochemical composition of tissues changes with age; physiologic capacity decreases; the adaptive processes responsible for maintaining homoeostasis weaken; and an increased susceptibility and vulnerability to disease (Auerhahn et al., 2007). The rate at which these changes occur is different for different organs and tissues and varies from individual to individual (AGS, 2002). An overview of some of the normal physical changes of aging is presented in Table 3.2.

Normal physical changes of aging is one of the most important areas of gerontological content that needs to be included in APN programs whose graduates will provide care to older adults. APNs who deliver care to older adults must be able to differentiate the normal physical changes of aging from pathological changes due to disease. They also need to be aware of the impact that these changes of aging have on the presentation of illness and response to treatment.

TABLE 3.2. Normal Physical Changes of Aging

System	Physical Changes
Bones and joints	Bones become less dense. Intervertebral discs become thinner. Joint cartilage thins. Ligaments and tendons become less elastic.
Muscles and body fat	Muscle mass and strength decrease. The percentage of body fat increases and the distribution changes.
Eyes	The lenses stiffen, become denser, and yellow. Pupils react more slowly to changes in light. Number of nerve cells decreases. The eyes produce less fluid, making them feel dry.
Ears	Hearing high-pitched sounds becomes more difficult. Ear wax, which interferes with hearing, tends to accumulate more.
Mouth and nose	Taste buds on the tongue decrease in number and sensitivity. Saliva production decreases. Gums recede slightly and tooth enamel tends to wear away. Lining of the nose becomes thinner and drier, and the nerve endings in the nose deteriorate. Nose tends to lengthen and thin, and the tip tends to droop.
Skin	Skin becomes thinner, less elastic, drier, and finely wrinkled. Fat layer under the skin thins. Number of nerve endings, sweat glands, and blood vessels in the skin decreases. Number of melanocytes decreases.
Brain and nervous system	Number of nerve cells and receptors in the brain decreases. Number of cells in the spinal cord begins to decrease. Blood flow to the brain decreases.
Heart and blood vessels	Heart and blood vessels become stiffer leading to a tendency for an increase in blood pressure. Despite these changes, a normal older heart functions well.
Lungs	The diaphragm tends to weaken. The number of alveoli and capillaries in the lungs decreases. Lungs become less elastic.

TABLE 3.2. Normal Physical Changes of Aging (*Continued*)

System	Physical Changes
Digestive system	The digestive system is less affected by aging than other systems. Lactase production may decrease. Transit time through the large intestine may slow. The number of liver cells decreases and blood flow through the liver slows.
Kidneys and urinary tract	The number of kidney cells decreases. Blood flow through the kidneys decreases. Bladder volume decreases and bladder muscles weaken. In women, the urethra shortens and its lining becomes thinner. In men, the prostate gland tends to enlarge.
Reproductive organs	The effects of aging on sex hormone levels are more obvious in women than in men. Ovaries and uterus shrink. Vaginal tissues become thinner, drier, and less elastic. Breasts become less firm and more fibrous. In men, testosterone levels decrease gradually. Blood flow to the penis decreases.
Endocrine system	The levels and activity of some endocrine hormones decrease but will have no noticeable effect on older adults. Insulin is less effective and production may decrease.
Blood production	Amount of active bone marrow decreases but can usually produce enough blood cells throughout life.
Immune system	Cells of the immune system act more slowly.

Source: Porter, R. S., Kaplan, J. L., & Homeier, B. P. (Eds.). (2009). Older people's health issues: Changes in the body. *Merck Manual Online Medical Library* (Home ed.). Retrieved from http://www.merck.com/mmhe/sec26/ch320/ch320b.html#sec26-ch320-ch320b-156#sec26-ch320-ch320b-156

PSYCHOSOCIAL NEEDS

A discussion of the inclusion of gerontological content about psychosocial needs in APN educational programs must begin with the psychosocial and developmental theories of aging. There are numerous psychosocial theories of aging, such as Disengagement, Activity, Continuity, Role Theory, Social Exchange, Modernization, Age Stratification Theory, and Person-environment Fit Theory (Edelman & Mandle, 2006), with varying degrees of evidence to support them. The group of developmental theories, including those of Erickson, Peck, Maslow, and Jung, speak to the need for successful completion of developmental tasks throughout the life span including old age. Like the theories of physical aging discussed earlier, the psychosocial and developmental theories of aging contribute to the scientific basis of care of older adults.

Older adults face a multitude of psychosocial stressors. These include major life events such as retirement, loss of a spouse or other loved one, remarriage, and changes in living arrangements including relocation. There are also those that occur on a daily or regular basis such as caregiver burden, social isolation, depression, physical and chemical restraint, and elder mistreatment. The potential for loss of function and independence is another major stressor for many older adults (Porter, Kaplan, & Homeier, 2009).

Coping strategies of older adults have been studied extensively. There are a group of coping strategies that older adults frequently use that are based on the premise of reframing their performance in order to gain positive reinforcement and improved self-esteem. For example, an older adult selects activities in which he or she is likely to succeed and reframes the definition of success by a comparison of his or her performance to that of other older adults instead of performance at a younger age. As an adult ages, he or she develops compensatory strategies that will allow continued success. Other successful coping strategies for older adults are social involvement, social networks, spiritual or religious involvement, and healthy behaviors. Social involvement strengthens the older adult's connection to the community and serves to confirm his or her value to the community. Strong social networks have been shown to reduce morbidity and mortality, strengthen self-efficacy, and moderate age-related stress. Spiritual or religious involvement and healthy behaviors have both been shown to have a positive relationship with health and well-being (Auerhahn et al., 2007).

It is important for APN students to have an understanding of the psychosocial issues of older adults and their impact on the total picture of health and well-being. This content will provide valuable information for their enhanced understanding of the holistic context within which APNs treat their patients.

HEALTH PROMOTION

Health promotion can be defined as a combination of educational and environmental supports for actions and conditions of living conducive to health. Its primary purpose is to enable people to gain greater control over the determinants of their own health through individual control and community decisions and actions. Older adults are the fastest growing segment of our population. Most of them live in the community with only a small percentage residing in nursing homes. The focus for the majority of older adults is functional independence, which for them defines quality of life. Health promotion for older adults has been proven to work on improving health status (Haber, 2010). It can and should be a priority for older adults.

Content that needs to be included in APN programs that prepare graduates to care for older adults should focus on the identification of social and lifestyle risk factors that can affect the health and well-being of older adults (Federal Interagency Forum, 2008; Towner, 2006). Knowledge of the different levels of prevention strategies and their goals is also essential (AGS, 2002). Primary prevention strategies are designed to maximize functional independence. Secondary and tertiary prevention strategies focus on early identification of disease and reduction of morbidity and mortality, respectively. It is important to include content that stresses that the focus of prevention programs for older adults should be on health needs that are common to older adults, such as immunization, prevention of falls, social support, emotional support, and intellectual stimulation (Bradshaw & Klein, 2007). And that it is also important to consider functional status, life expectancy, personal preference, and goals of care (Leipzig et al., 2009).

Health promotion is an expected part of APN practice (National Association of Clinical Nurse Specialists [NACNS], 2004; National Organization of Nurse Practitioners Faculties [NONPF], 2006). As such, it is essential that content related to health promotion of the older adult be included in APN educational programs that prepare graduates to care for older adults.

DIAGNOSIS AND MANAGEMENT OF EPISODIC, ACUTE, AND CHRONIC ILLNESS

The overall approach to the diagnosis and management of episodic, acute, and chronic illness in the older adult needs to first consider the impact of age-related changes on the presentation of illness and the ability to distinguish normal aging from pathology. Second is the recognition of conditions that present almost exclusively in older adulthood, such as polymyalgia rheumatica and pseudogout, and those conditions that have altered presentations in elderly patients, such as pneumonia, diabetes, thyroid disease, myocardial infarction, rheumatoid arthritis, and gout

(Beck, 2006; Ham, Sloane, Warshaw, Bernard, & Flaherty, 2006). Finally, unique to older adults are the geriatric syndromes that frequently contribute to the development of or are a result of a change in overall function, and are the key to an impending, often reversible, condition that needs attention. Careful management if not prevention of geriatric syndromes is critical to enhancing overall quality of life of older adults.

Components of Comprehensive Geriatric Assessment

The approach to geriatric assessment is generally considered to be multidimensional, often involving the input of other members of a geriatric interdisciplinary team. The ability to collect all components of a comprehensive geriatric assessment takes time and usually is completed over a series of visits if completed by the independent provider. In the hospitalized setting, this complete assessment often is limited to patients with multiple medical problems and functional impairments. APNs benefit by using standardized instruments not only to obtain baseline data, but also to compare findings when there is a change in the patient's status. Using common standardized instruments also facilitates communication among health care providers. The components of a comprehensive geriatric assessment include: functional ability, cognitive and mental status, socioenvironmental situations (including family and caregiver support), and often nutritional status (Beers, Jones, Berkwitts, Kaplan, & Porter, 2000).

The assessment of the older adult also needs to incorporate all other aspects of a conventional medical history, with special attention paid to the unique nature of this population. Discerning the chief complaint of an older adult may be complicated due to the fact that older adults have a tendency to underreport symptoms based on fear, acceptance of the condition as a result of old age, and cognitive impairments (Kennedy-Malone, Fletcher, & Plank, 2003). Compounding the complexity of illness management in older adults is the frequent presentation of concomitant symptoms, chronic conditions, and polypharmacy including self-medication.

Past medical history needs to be thorough, highlighting on prior presentation of illness, treatment of exacerbations of conditions, and response to medical regimens. Astute health care providers need to uncover any situations that led to noncompliance in the past. A family history of an older adult needs to address conditions that occurred in parents and siblings in later life, especially any malignancies and neurodegenerative conditions, as well as cause of death. Information collected as part of the social history should not overlook habits such as alcohol, tobacco, or use of illicit drugs. Sexual history and physical activity levels need to be evaluated to determine if there is a change in status due to health conditions.

The process for collecting relevant data for the review of systems and physical examination of the older adult is similar to that of a younger person, once the health care provider considers the impact of normal aging to include sensory impairments, memory loss, and concomitant symptoms. Information contained in Table 3.3 serves as a guide for collecting a review of systems and physical examination on an older adult that is so critical for making an accurate diagnosis.

There are few gold standards in diagnostics for older adults that often lead to false positives and negatives, such as when serum antibodies or the erythrocyte sedimentation rate is evaluated. It is advantageous that APNs are familiar with common laboratory values for older adults and apply the adjusted values when diagnosing medical conditions (Kennedy-Malone et al., 2003). Additionally, the average older adult takes four to five prescription medications a day and, because drugs are metabolized more slowly and their effects are more prolonged in the body in older adults, side effects from medications can occur that are often mistaken for a new disease presentation (Auerhahn et al., 2007).

ATYPICAL PRESENTATION OF ILLNESS

A challenge to managing the care of older adults is the ability to recognize altered, atypical, and nonspecific disease presentation (Cassel, Leipzig, Cohen, Larson, & Meier, 2003; Ham et al., 2006). Vague, blunted, and delayed symptomatology that differs from common disease presentation in younger adults is often overlooked or diagnosed only when complications ensue (Meiner & Lueckenotte, 2005). Often the progression of the condition is insidious and presents as an abrupt change of function and/or alteration in cognition. Recognizing signal signs of atypical and altered presentations is critical to prevent morbidity and mortality. In addition to functional decline and alteration in cognition, other key signs and symptoms include: fatigue, weakness, anorexia, immobility, incontinence, falls, altered pain perception, dyspnea, tachypnea, and altered ability to develop a temperature (Ham et al., 2006). Table 3.4 depicts common conditions that present in older adults with an atypical presentation.

TABLE 3.3. Geriatric History and Physical Considerations

System of the Body	Special Problems Pertinent to Older Adults
Head, eyes, ears, nose, and throat	*History:* Visual changes, alteration in color perception, scotomas, floaters, sensitivity to glare, difficulty with night driving and depth perception, lack of peripheral vision, lack of central vision, cloudiness, diplopia, hearing loss, vertigo, tinnitus, alteration or lack of sense of smell, and decreased saliva
	Physical: Changes in visual acuity, ptosis, proptosis, entropion and ectropion eyelids, cataracts, fundoscopic changes such as cotton-wool patches, cerumen impaction, caries, periodontal disease, tooth decay, tooth loss, oral-pharyngeal cancers, and xerostomia
Integumentary	*History:* Exposure to irritants, history of extended exposure to sun, extended immobility, and alterations in temperature
	Physical: Xerosis, lesions, rashes, pressure ulcers, skin tears, discoloration, ulceration, and erysipelas
Cardiovascular	*History:* Fatigue, chest pain, palpitations, syncope, irregular heartbeats, confusion, and diaphoresis
	Physical: Carotid bruits, arrhythmias, abnormal heart sounds, peripheral edema, absent or weak pulses, elevated pulse pressure, and orthostatic hypotension
Respiratory	*History:* Dyspnea, orthopnea, chronic cough, chest discomfort, night sweats, and low-grade fevers
	Physical: Rales, hypoxia, wheezing, and hemoptysis
Gastrointestinal	*History:* Dentition problems, anorexia, constipation, diarrhea, fecal incontinence, regurgitation, dysphagia, globus, hoarseness, bloating, and abdominal pain
	Physical: Abdominal masses, bruits, weight loss, fecal occult blood, hemorrhoids, and fissures
Genitourinary	*History:* Nocturia, incontinence, bacteriuria, overactive bladder, sexual dysfunction to include erectile dysfunction and vaginal atrophy and dryness
	Physical: Cystocele, rectocele, prolapsed uterus, anal sphincter tone
Musculoskeletal	*History:* Interference with physical function due to pain or range of motion, swelling, and erythema
	Physical: Kyphosis, gibbous, joint and periarticular tenderness, swelling, nodularity, crepitation, limitation of movement, muscle atrophy, fractures, and contractures

TABLE 3.3. Geriatric History and Physical Considerations *(Continued)*

System of the Body	Special Problems Pertinent to Older Adults
Neurological	*History:* Sleep disorders, dizziness, new onset of headaches, memory loss, paralysis, paresthesia, loss of consciousness, seizures, pain especially associated with loss of function, and impaired judgment
	Physical: Alterations in sensation, proprioception, evidence of tremors, fasciculations, gait disorders, reduction in strength, slowness in movement, rigidity, changes in reflexes, and increased time to perform and learn tasks
Metabolic/endocrine	*History:* Alterations in temperature, fatigue, frequent infections, dehydration, weakness, drug-induced illness, and malnutrition
	Physical: Pallor, weakness, and weight loss or gain
Psychosocial	*History:* Depression, grief, loneliness, dependency, and end-of-life issues
	Physical: Geriatric depression scale, tests of cognition, alcohol abuse scales, social support indexes, elder abuse and neglect tools

Source: American Academy of Family Physicians (AAFP). (2008). *Recommended curriculum guidelines for family medicine residents: Care of older adults.* Retrieved from http://www.aafp.org/online/etc/medialib/aafp_org/documents/about/rap/curriculum/olderadults. Par.0001.File.tmp/Reprint264.pdf.
Source: Beck, J. C. (2006). *Geriatric review syllabus: A core curriculum in geriatric medicine* (6th ed.). New York: American Geriatrics Society.
Source: Ham, R. J., Sloane, P. D.,Warshaw, G. A., Bernard, M. A., & Flaherty, E. (Eds.). (2006). *Primary care geriatrics: A case-based approach* (5th ed.). St. Louis, MO: Mosby.
Source: Kennedy-Malone, L., Fletcher, K. R., & Plank, L. M. (2003). *Management guidelines for nurse practitioners caring for older adults* (2nd ed.). Philadelphia: F. A. Davis.

GERIATRIC SYNDROMES

"Presentation of illness in older persons is less often a single, specific symptom or sign, which in younger patients announces the organ with pathology. Older persons often present with nonspeficific problems that are in fact functional deficits. . . . These deficits have been named geriatric syndromes" (Cassel et al., 2003, p. 152). Geriatric syndromes are also thought to be multifactorial, resulting in a single phenomenology (Flacker, 2003). Older adults present with conditions that generally have more than one cause and involve multiple body systems, often contributing to functional

TABLE 3.4. Altered Presentation of Illness in Older Adults

Illness	Atypical Presentations
Infectious diseases	Absence of fever Sepsis without usual leukocytosis and fever Falls, decreased appetite or fluid intake, confusion, and change in functional status
"Silent" acute abdomen	Absence of symptoms (silent presentation) Mild discomfort and constipation Some tachypnea and possibly vague respiratory symptoms
"Silent malignancy"	Back pain secondary to metastases from slow-growing breast masses Silent masses of the bowel
"Silent" myocardial infarction	Absence of chest pain Vague symptoms of fatigue, nausea, and a decrease in functional status Classic presentations: shortness of breath, more common complaint than chest pain
Nondyspneic pulmonary edema	May not subjectively experience the classic symptoms such as paroxysmal nocturnal dyspnea or coughing Typical onset is insidious with changes in function, food or fluid intake, or confusion
Thyroid disease	Hyperthyroidism presenting as "apathetic thyrotoxicosis," i.e., fatigue and a slowing down Hypothyroidism and presenting with confusion and agitation
Depression	Lack of sadness Somatic complaints, such as appetite changes, vague GI symptoms, constipation, and sleep disturbances Hyperactivity Sadness misinterpreted by provider as normal consequences of aging Medical problems that mask depression
Medical illness that presents as depression	Hypo- and hyperthyroid disease that presents as diminished energy and apathy

Source: Adapted from Ham, R. J., Sloane, P. D., Warshaw, G. A., Bernard, M. A., & Flaherty, E. (Eds.). (2006). Primary care geriatrics: A case-based approach (5th ed., p. 29). St. Louis, MO: Mosby. Reprinted with permission of the publisher, Elsevier Inc.

disability. Commonly identified geriatric syndromes include: dementia, delirium, falls, incontinence, failure to thrive, sleep disorders, immobility, malnutrition, dysphagia, and pain. A comprehensive assessment is usually warranted when a patient presents with one or more of these syndromes. Resolution of a reversible geriatric syndrome often leads to improvement in overall function (Cassel et al., 2003). While geriatric syndromes often involve multiple body systems, strategies to incorporate many of these syndromes into a particular body system are addressed in Chapter 9.

SUMMARY

In order to ensure the competency of APNs caring for older adults, the gerontological content identified in this chapter, while extensive, needs to be integrated across the APN curriculum. This chapter presented a detailed overview of specific areas that should be addressed in NP and CNS programs whose graduates will provide care to older adults. It is by no means totally inclusive. Subsequent chapters will provide content designed to enable nongerontological APN faculty to accomplish the task of integrating gerontological content into their curricula. Chapters 4 and 5 present detailed lists of print media and Internet resources, respectively. Chapter 6 discusses a competency-based framework and is followed by three chapters that offer guidance for the integration of gerontological content into the graduate nursing core, APN core, and specialty courses. The last chapter consists of a series of "success stories" written by faculty who teach in APN programs and who have successfully integrated gerontological content into nongerontological APN courses.

REFERENCES

Administration on Aging, U.S. Dept. of Health and Human Services (AOA). (2008) *A profile of older Americans: 2008.* Retrieved from http://www.aoa.gov/AoARoot/Index.aspx

American Academy of Family Physicians (AAFP). (2008). *Recommended curriculum guidelines for family medicine residents: Care of older adults.* Retrieved from http://www.aafp.org/online/etc/medialib/aafp_org/documents/about/rap/curriculum/olderadults.Par.0001.File.tmp/Reprint264.pdf

American Geriatrics Society (AGS). (2002). *Areas of basic competency for the care of older patients for medical and osteopathic schools.* Retrieved from http://www.americangeriatrics.org/education/competency.shtml

American Geriatrics Society Education Committee (AGS). (2004). *Curriculum guidelines for geriatrics training in internal medicine residency programs.* Retrieved from http://www.americangeriatrics.org/education/resident.shtml

Auerhahn, C., Capezuti, E., Flaherty, E., & Resnick, B. (Eds.). (2007). *Geriatric nursing review syllabus: A core curriculum in advanced practice geriatric nursing* (2nd ed.). New York: American Geriatrics Society.

Beck, J. C. (2006). *Geriatric review syllabus: A core curriculum in geriatric medicine* (6th ed.). New York: American Geriatrics Society.

Beers, M. H., Jones, T. V., Berkwitts, M., Kaplan, J. L., & Porter, R. S. (Eds.). (2000). Comprehensive geriatric assessment. *The Merck Manual of Geriatrics* (3rd ed.). Retrieved from http://www.merck.com/mkgr/mmg/sec1/ch4/ch4a.jsp

Bradshaw, J., & Klein, W. C. (2007). Health promotion. In J. Blackburn & C. Dulmus (Eds.), *Handbook of gerontology, evidence-based approaches to theory, practice, and policy.* Hoboken, NJ: John Wiley & Sons.

Cassel, C. K., Leipzig, R. M., Cohen, H. J., Larson, E. B., & Meier, D. E. (Eds.). (2003). *Geriatric medicine: An evidence-based approach* (4th ed.). New York: Springer.

Cummings, S. M., & Galambos, C. (2002). Predictors of graduate social work students' interest in aging-related work. *Journal of Gerontological Social Work, 39,* 77–94.

Edelman, C. L., & Mandle, C. L. (2006). *Health promotion throughout the life span* (6th ed.). St. Louis: Mosby.

Federal Interagency Forum on Aging-Related Statistics (Federal Interagency Forum). (2008). *Older Americans 2008: Key indicators of well-being.* Washington, DC: U.S. Government Printing Office.

Flacker, J. M. (2003). What is a geriatric syndrome anyway? *Journal of the American Geriatrics Society, 51,* 574–573.

Haber, D. (2010). *Health promotion and aging: Practical applications for health professionals* (5th ed.). New York: Springer Publishing Company.

Ham, R. J., Sloane, P. D., Warshaw, G. A., Bernard, M. A., & Flaherty, E. (Eds.). (2006). *Primary care geriatrics: A case-based approach* (5th ed.). St. Louis, MO: Mosby.

Kennedy-Malone, L., Fletcher, K. R., & Plank, L. M. (2003). *Management guidelines for nurse practitioners caring for older adults* (2nd ed.). Philadelphia: F. A. Davis.

Kennedy-Malone, L., Penrod, J., Kohlenberg, E. M., Letvak, S. A., Crane, P. B., Tesh, A., Kolanowski, A., Hupcey, J., & Milone-Nuzzo, P. (2006). Integrating gerontology competencies into graduate nursing programs. *Journal of Professional Nursing, 22*(2), 123–128.

Kite, M. E., & Wagner, L. S. (2004). Attitudes toward older adults. In T. D. Nelson (Ed.), *Ageism: Stereotyping and prejudice against older persons* (pp. 129–162). Cambridge, MA: MIT Press.

Kohlenberg, E., Kennedy-Malone, L., Crane, P., & Letvak, S. (2007). Infusing gerontological nursing content into advanced practice nursing education. *Nursing Outlook, 55,* 38–43.

Leipzig, R. M., Granville, L, Simpson, D., Anderson, M. B., et al. (2009). Keeping granny safe on July 1: A consensus on minimum geriatrics competencies for graduating medical students. *Academic Medicine, 84*(5), 604–610.

Meiner, S., & Lueckenotte, A. (2005) *Gerontological nursing* (3rd ed.). St. Louis, MO: Mosby.

Morley, J. E. (2006). Sexuality and aging. In M. S. J. Pathy, A. J. Sinclair, & J. E. Morley (Eds.), *Principles and practice of geriatric medicine* (4th ed.). Hoboken, NJ: John Wiley & Sons, Ltd.

National Association of Clinical Nurse Specialists. (2004). *Statement on Clinical Nurse Specialist Practice and Education* (2nd ed.). Harrisburg, PA: Author.

National Organization of Nurse Practitioner Faculties and the American Association of Colleges of Nursing. (2006). *Domains and Core Competencies of Nurse Practitioner Practice.* Washington, DC: Author.

Nelson, T. D. (2005). Ageism: Prejudice against our feared future self. *Journal of Social Issues, 61*(2), 207–221.

Newell, D. A., Raji, M., Lieberman, S., & Beach, R. E. (2004). Integrating geriatric content into a medical school curriculum: Description of a successful model. *Gerontology and Geriatrics Education, 25*(2), 15–32.

Perlman, R. M. (2003). Commemorating the 50th anniversary of JAGS: The aging syndrome. *Journal of the American Geriatrics Society, 51*(4), 558–561.

Porter, R. S., Kaplan, J. L., & Homeier, B. P. (Eds.). (2009). Older people's health issues: Changes in the body. *Merck Manual Online Medical Library* (Home ed.). Retrieved from http://www.merck.com/mmhe/sec26/ch320/ch320b. html#sec26-ch320-ch320b-156#sec26-ch320-ch320b-156

Rosen, A. L., Zlotnik, J. L., Curl, A. L., & Green, R. G. (2000). *CSWE SAGE-SW National Competencies Survey and Report.* Retrieved from http://www.cswe.org/18949.aspx?catGroupId=6&catId=77

Ryan, M., & McCauley, D. (2004/2005). We built it and they did not come: Knowledge and attitudes of baccalaureate nursing students toward the elderly. *Journal of the New York State Nurses Association, 35,* 5–9.

Thornlow, D. K., Auerhahn, C., & Stanley, J. (2006). A necessity not a luxury: Preparing advanced practice nurses to care for older adults. *Journal of Professional Nursing, 22,* 116–122.

Towner, E. M. (2006). Assessment of geriatric knowledge: An online tool for appraising entering APN students. *Journal of Professional Nursing, 22*(2), 112–115.

Wesley, S. C. (2005). Enticing students to careers in gerontology: Faculty and student perspectives. *Gerontology and Geriatrics Education, 25,* 13–29.

World Health Organization (WHO). (1999). *Ageing: Exploding the myths.* Retrieved from http://whqlibdoc.who.int/hq/1999/WHO_HSC_AHE_99.1.pdf

Resources for Integration of Gerontological Content Into Advanced Practice Nursing Curriculum

CHAPTER 4

Print Media Resources for Integration of Gerontological Content Into Advanced Practice Nursing Curriculum

Carolyn Auerhahn

There are a number of challenges facing APN faculty when trying to include gerontological content in nongerontological APN courses. In addition to those discussed in Chapter 2, a major challenge for some faculty is the lack of knowledge about available resources for gerontological content. If this knowledge deficit is present, even the best-intentioned APN faculty member will find the work of integration of gerontological content into nongerontological courses daunting.

This chapter will present an annotated list of selected print media resources for gerontological/geriatric content. The collection of texts and journals highlighted in this chapter were selected based on their relevance to APN education and the care of older adults. They represent the work of multiple disciplines including nursing, medicine, and social work. The majority are evidence-based and were published within the last two years. Sources used in the selection process included the bookshelves of the author, recommendations from other gerontological APN faculty, and the Internet. It is by no means intended to be an all-inclusive list, but will provide APN faculty with an arsenal with which to begin the task.

The chapter is divided into two sections: Selected Geriatric Text Resources and Selected Geriatric Journals. The texts have been further organized into five categories: comprehensive, health promotion, assessment, primary care, and acute and long-term care. For each of the texts and journals, a brief description regarding intended audience, content, and availability is included. Also included is an assessment of the appropriateness of the resource for APN students.

SELECTED GERIATRIC TEXT RESOURCES

Comprehensive

Geriatric Nursing Review Syllabus: A Core Curriculum in Advanced Practice Geriatric Nursing, Second Edition

The *Geriatric Nursing Review Syllabus: A Core Curriculum in Advanced Practice Geriatric Nursing*, Second Edition (*GNRS2*), is a concise, comprehensive text developed specifically for APN education by the American Geriatrics Society, in collaboration with the Hartford Institute for Geriatric Nursing at New York University College of Nursing (HIGN). The editors, all of whom are expert gerontological APNs, have adapted the content in the *Geriatrics Review Syllabus: A Core Curriculum in Geriatric Medicine*, Sixth Edition (*GRS6*), to more accurately represent APN practice in the care of older adults (Auerhahn, Capezuti, Flaherty, & Resnick, 2007). Content relevant to the APN approach to care of older adults, the "value-added" components of APN practice, and references specific to APN content and practice were added as indicated. It is a respected source for content on the care of older adults and an excellent teaching resource for the integration of gerontological content into all APN educational programs.

GNRS2 is an evidence-based text consisting of 59 chapters divided into the following five sections: Current Issues in Aging; Approach to the Patient; Syndromes; Psychiatry; and Diseases and Disorders. Topics included in the Current Issues on Aging section include demographics, biology of aging, psychosocial issues, legal and ethical issues, and financing, coverage, and costs of health care. Approach to the Patient includes assessment, cultural aspects of care, physical activity, prevention, pharmacotherapy, complementary and alternative medicine, elder mistreatment, hospital care, perioperative care, rehabilitation, nursing home care, community-based care, palliative care, and persistent pain. In the Syndromes section, the syndromes included are visual impairment, hearing impairment, dizziness, syncope, malnutrition, eating and feeding problems, urinary incontinence, gait impairment, falls, osteoporosis, dementia, behavior problems in dementia, delirium, sleep problems, and pressure ulcers. The Psychiatry section includes depression and other mood disorders, anxiety, psychotic, personality, and somatoform disorders, substance abuse, and mental retardation. The section, Diseases and Disorders, covers all of the body systems with separate chapters on hypertension, diabetes mellitus, disorders of sexual function, prostate disease, and oncology. References at the end of each chapter provide a resource for further exploration of the topics. There is also an appendix that contains material that is useful for APN practice, such as guidelines for anticoagulation, the Geriatric Depression Scale, and a nutrition screening tool.

In addition to the content described above, there are 100 case-oriented multiple choice questions with answers and critiques that have also been adapted for APN practice. These questions are intended solely for use as a self-assessment program and not for use as practice test questions for the Gerontological NP certification examinations administered by the American Nurses Credentialing Center and the American Academy of Nurse Practitioners.

The editors of *GNRS2* are Carolyn Auerhahn, EdD, ANP, GNP-BC, FAANP; Elizabeth Capezuti, PhD, RN, FAAN; Ellen Flaherty, PhD, GNP-BC; and Barbara Resnick, PhD, CRNP, FAAN, FAANP. The *GNRS2* is available only from the American Geriatrics Society and can be ordered at www.americangeriatrics.org/products.

Geriatrics at Your Fingertips

Geriatrics at Your Fingertips (GAYF) is an indispensable resource for all health care professionals who provide care to older adults. It is available in a pocket-sized, print version and a downloadable PDA version. Updated annually, it provides the user with instant access to current vital clinical information related to the care of older adults across all health care settings. It is a collaborative, interprofessional publication authored by experts in geriatric medicine, gerontological nursing, and geriatric pharmacy.

Content in the 2009 *GAYF* consists of up-to-date clinical guidelines, diagnostic strategies, management choices, and information on state-of-the-art medications, with specific content related to prescribing for older adults. Disease-specific content covers all body systems with separate chapters on dementia, depression, osteoporosis, and pain. There are separate chapters addressing the geriatric syndromes such as falls, malnutrition, and incontinence. Also included are chapters on assessment, prevention, women's health, and sexual dysfunction. The appendix contains assessment tools, guidelines on unnecessary drug use in nursing homes, information about Medicare Part D, and a list of useful Web sites and important phone numbers for both providers and patients. The content in *GAYF* is presented in an outline format with tables, algorithms, and diagrams, in combination with a detailed subject and medication index, makes it easy to locate information quickly.

The authors of the 2009 *GAYF* are David Reuben, MD; Keela A. Herr, PhD, RN; James T. Pacala, MD, MS; Bruce G. Pollock, MD, PhD; Jane F. Potter, MD; and Todd P. Semla, MS, PharmD. *GAYF* is published by the American Geriatrics Society and, as noted, is updated annually. It can only be purchased online and the latest version can be ordered at www.americangeriatrics.org/products.

Essentials of Clinical Geriatrics, Sixth Edition

Essentials of Clinical Geriatrics, Sixth Edition, presents a comprehensive summary of the essential issues in the care of older adults and offers realistic advice for the diagnosis and management of the most frequently encountered health problems in this population. Included in the text are numerous tables that summarize the content and an appendix of Internet resources related to the care of older adults. In addition, unlike earlier editions of this text where the authors consisted only of experts in geriatric medicine, this edition has added a gerontological NP as an author, thereby providing a wider perspective on care of older adults. Another addition to this edition is an evidence-based summary at the end of selected chapters. The *Essentials of Clinical Geriatrics* has long been regarded as one of the leading textbooks for clinical care of older adults. Its availability as a paperback, its format, and the changes made in this edition make it a worthwhile clinical reference for APNs in all settings.

The *Essentials of Clinical Geriatrics*, Sixth Edition, is divided into three parts: Part I: The Aging Patient and Geriatric Assessment; Part II: Differential Diagnosis and Management; and Part III: General Management Strategies. The first part presents information related to the care of older adults with regard to the aging process, demography, epidemiology, health services utilization, assessment, and principles of management of chronic disease. Part II on Differential Diagnosis and Management includes chapters on prevention and common health care problems found in this population, specifically confusion, depression, incontinence, falls, and immobility. Part III focuses on General Management Strategies for cardiovascular problems, conditions that can lead to decreased vitality, and sensory impairment. Also included in this part are chapters on drug therapy, health services, nursing home care, and ethical issues for older adults.

The authors of the *Essentials of Clinical Geriatrics*, Sixth Edition, are Robert L. Kane, MD; Joseph G. Ouslander, MD; Itmar B. Abrass, MD; and Barbara Resnick, PhD, CRNP, FAAN, FAANP. It is published by McGraw-Hill Professional Publishing Company, and available in paperback only.

Hazzard's Geriatric Medicine & Gerontology, Sixth Edition

Hazzard's Geriatric Medicine & Gerontology, Sixth Edition, is a comprehensive, evidence-based text that encompasses all areas of gerontology and clinical geriatrics. Formerly known as *Principles of Geriatric Medicine & Gerontology*, it differs greatly from previous editions. There is a global, multidisciplinary perspective to this edition, reflected by both the geographical and multidisciplinary composition of the contributing authors. Clinical practice guidelines and references to other hallmarks of evidence-based practice are more manifest in this edition. There are new chapters that focus on inflammation and aging, emergency geriatrics, transitions of care, social work, rural aging, and international geriatric care. There are also three new chapters, Principles of Pharmacology, Psychoactive Drug Therapy, and Appropriate Antibiotic Use, which address pharmacological management of the older adult. A major change in the sixth edition is its availability, in addition to its print format, as an online version accessible through McGraw-Hill's Access Medicine Web site. The changes in perspective, content, and authorship in *Hazzard's Geriatric Medicine & Gerontology*, Sixth Edition, acknowledge the heterogeneity of the geriatric health care team making it relevant for use by a wider range of health care professionals. The online version not only makes it more accessible, but facilitates the continuation of the text's state-of-the-art reputation by allowing for ongoing updates. In addition, APN faculty and students at academic institutions that subscribe to Access Medicine will have free online access to this text.

Hazzard's Geriatric Medicine & Gerontology, Sixth Edition, consists of 130 chapters divided into four parts: Principles of Gerontology, Principles of Geriatrics, Geriatric Syndromes, and Organ Systems and Diseases. The content in Part I: Principles of Gerontology is focused on the science, demography, epidemiology, and psychosocial aspects of aging. It also includes content on general principles of pharmacology and strategies for health promotion and disease prevention. Part II: Principles of Geriatrics covers topics that are integral to the clinical care of older adults, such as assessment, organization of health care and health care settings, nutrition, sensory function, and sexuality. There is also a chapter on special management issues such as complementary and alternative medicine, self-management, palliative care, and legal and ethical issues. Aging and homeostatic regulation, frailty, delirium, falls, sleep disorders, dizziness, syncope, pressure ulcers, incontinence, and elder mistreatment are discussed in Part III: Geriatric Syndromes. The last part of the text is divided into sections by body systems. The first chapter in each of these sections is a discussion of the changes in that system due to the aging process. Subsequent chapters in each section deal with health needs and diseases and disorders that are prevalent in older adults.

The editors of *Hazzard's Geriatric Medicine & Gerontology*, Sixth Edition, are Jeffrey B. Halter, MD; Joseph G. Ouslander, MD; Mary E. Tinetti, MD; Stephanie Studenski, MD, MPH; Kevin P. High, MD, MS; and Sanjay Asthana, MD. It is published by McGraw-Hill in a print and online version.

Health Promotion

Health Promotion and Aging: Practical Applications for Health Professionals, Fifth Edition

Health Promotion and Aging: Practical Applications for Health Professionals, Fifth Edition, is a comprehensive text about health promotion and aging written for all health care professionals. Trained as a sociologist with a specialty in gerontology, the author David Haber has spent his career developing and evaluating community-based health promotion projects for older adults. This newest edition of *Health Promotion and Aging: Practical Applications for Health Professionals* has undergone substantial revision. Several new content areas and terms have been added such as Social Networking, Brain Games, Mental Health Parity, Wii Habilitation, and Sleep-Related Medical Disorders. Other additions include learning outcomes and questions for consideration in each chapter. It has an evidence-based focus and a concentration on practical applications. The practical nature of the text is supported by the inclusion of assessment and health promotion tools, resource lists, checklists, and tables. Earlier editions of *Health Promotion and*

Aging: Practical Applications for Health Professionals have been highly respected for their advocacy for health promotion of older adults. This new edition continues the legacy of those that came before with its innovative and timely additions. It is one of only a few health promotion texts focused on older adults and its emphasis on practical application makes it ideal for use in APN education and practice.

In addition to the new content areas already discussed, the fifth edition contains updated versions of all content areas found in earlier versions. Topics include background information on economic, political, social, environmental, and ethical issues relevant to older adults. Several chapters focus on health promotion and health behavior, and include the basics such as exercise, nutrition, weight management, and smoking. The chapter on clinical preventive services includes content on the controversy surrounding screening and prophylaxis. There are also chapters on communication and collaboration with older adults, complementary and alternative medicine, diversity, social support, community health, and public health.

David Haber, PhD, is the author of *Health Promotion and Aging: Practical Applications for Health Professionals*, Fifth Edition. It is published by Springer Publishing Company.

Nursing for Wellness of Older Adults, Fifth Edition

Nursing for Wellness of Older Adults, Fifth Edition, is an evidence-based text that presents a holistically conceptualized approach to wellness for older adults. Utilizing the Functional Consequences Theory developed by the author, a gerontological CNS, case manager, and board-certified holistic APN, the text focuses on age-related changes and risk factors for both physiologic and psychosocial function in older adults. The fifth edition has been updated to integrate recent research and other evidence into all sections of the text. Features from earlier editions such as progressive case studies, critical thinking exercises, cultural considerations, assessment and intervention boxes, and learning objectives are still included. Additions to the fifth edition include chapter highlights, clinical tool resources, and theory illustrations at the beginning of each chapter. A teaching and learning Internet package is available for use by both students and faculty. Although not written specifically for APN students, the holistic approach and nursing perspective of *Nursing for Wellness of Older Adults*, Fifth Edition, make it a useful reference for all nurses who provide care to older adults. The available

Internet resource package is a definite asset as well for both students and faculty.

Nursing for Wellness of Older Adults, Fifth Edition, consists of 29 chapters divided into five parts: Older Adults and Wellness; Nursing Considerations for Older Adults; Promoting Wellness in Psychosocial Function; Promoting Wellness in Physical Function; and Promoting Wellness in All Stages of Health and Illness. Part 1 presents the foundation for the text and includes the author's theoretical framework for the text, as well as theoretical perspectives on aging and culture and diversity of older adults. Consistent with its title, Part 2: Nursing Consideration for Older Adults focuses on relevant issues such as health care settings, medications, legal and ethical concerns, and elder mistreatment. Part 3 emphasizes cognitive and psychosocial function and includes delirium, depression, and dementia. Part 4 presents content about physical function essentially using a systems approach, as well as chapters on mobility and safety, sleep and rest, and thermoregulation. Content in the chapters in Parts 3 and 4 is presented within the context of the Functional Consequences Theory. Part 5 is a new addition to the text, and consists of three new chapters that deal with promoting wellness during illness, while experiencing pain and at the end of life.

Carol A. Miller, MSN, RN-BC, AHN-BC, is the author of *Nursing for Wellness of Older Adults*, Fifth Edition. It is published by Wolters Kluwer Health/Lippincott Williams & Wilkins.

Assessment

Handbook of Geriatric Assessment, Fourth Edition

The *Handbook of Geriatric Assessment*, Fourth Edition, is a text about the assessment of older adults written for use by physicians, nurse practitioners, social workers, researchers, and other health care professionals. It presents content and assessment tools that can be applied to a variety of settings and stresses the multidisciplinary nature of the geriatric assessment team. Its purpose, however, is not to be an all-inclusive manual of assessment tools, but rather to be an aid for use in the development of clinical assessment protocols. The editors and contributing authors are representative of the intended audience and come from the disciplines of medicine, nursing, social work, medical ethics, and public health. Because the content and assessment instruments presented are not site specific, it is an ideal reference for all APN students regardless of practice settings.

The *Handbook of Geriatric Assessment*, Fourth Edition, is organized into four sections: Section I: The Context of Assessment; Section II: Domains of Assessment; Section III: Settings of Assessment; and Section IV: Specialty Topics for Clinicians. Section I focuses on areas that may be relevant to other age groups but presents them from the perspective of providing care to older adults. These areas consist of emergency situations, ethnicity, driving, advance directives, mistreatment, and abuse. The second section presents content and assessment instruments for the eight domains representative of a multidimensional geriatric assessment that emphasize the prevention of functional decline: cognitive assessment; assessment for depression; substance use and abuse assessment; assessment of activities of daily living and instrumental activities of daily living; social assessment; physical assessment; pain assessment; and assessment for health promotion and disease prevention. Section III discusses assessment of older adults in their homes, in nursing homes, and at the time of hospitalization. The last section consists of three topics affecting the care of older adults that are reflective of the changing times in health care and in our society. These topics are compliance issues, interdisciplinary teams, and disaster preparedness.

Joseph J. Gallo, MD, MPH; Hillary R. Bogner, MD, MSCE; Terry Fulmer, PhD, RN, FAAN; and Gregory J. Paveza, MSW, PhD, are the editors of the *Handbook of Geriatric Assessment*, Fourth Edition. It is published by Jones and Bartlett Publishers.

Try This:® and *How to Try This* Series

The *Try This:*® series, also known as "Try This: Best Practices in Care for Older Adults," is an evidence-based series of assessment tools for use in the care of older adults. It is organized into three sections: a General Assessment; a Specialty Practice; and a Dementia Series. Each of these sections consists of easily understood, two-page documents written and edited by experts in gerontology. Each document provides an explanation of the importance of the topic being addressed, and an assessment tool that can be implemented in 20 minutes or less. The *How to Try This* series is a companion series to the *Try This:*® series. Developed by HIGN, in collaboration with the *American Journal of Nursing*, and with funding from the John A. Hartford Foundation, it consists of demonstration videos and corresponding print articles.

The General Assessment Series is composed of 30 issues consisting of assessment tools that include topics such as overall assessment, pressure ulcer risk, sleep quality, fall risk, and nutritional assessment. Three issues, Fulmer SPICES: An Overall Assessment Tool for Older Adults, Katz Index of Independence of Activities of Daily Living (ADL), and Mental Status Assessment of Older Adults: The Mini-Cog, are discussed here to provide examples from the series. Fulmer SPICES: An Overall Assessment Tool for Older Adults, created by Terry Fulmer, PhD, APRN, FAAN, in 1991 and most recently revised in 2007, is designed to obtain information about commonly occurring problems in older adults that may negatively impact their health status and functional ability. The acronym **SPICES** is derived from the problems addressed in the tool: Sleep disorders, Problems with eating or feeding, Incontinence, Confusion, Evidence of falls, and Skin breakdown and is an easy way to remember these common problems. It has been used extensively in hospital settings but may be used with healthy, community-dwelling older adults as well. The Katz Index of Independence of Activities of Daily Living (ADL) assesses the basic ADLs: bathing, dressing, toileting, transferring, incontinence, and feeding. It is widely regarded as the most appropriate tool to assess ADL functional status in older adults. Developed over 25 years ago, it has been used in a variety of settings for both baseline and periodic measurements. The Mental Status Assessment of Older Adults: The Mini-Cog issue provides a mental status screening tool that can be administered in 3 minutes, making it an ideal tool for use in all health care settings. The Mini-Cog consists of a three-item recall and the Clock Drawing Test, and has no bias related to education, culture, or language. It has been proven to be a valid and reliable tool for use in multiple clinical settings. A complete list of the issues in the General Assessment Series is included in Table 4.1. Also included in the table is a notation about which issue also includes a *How to Try This* companion.

The two remaining sections of the *Try This:®* series are the Specialty Practice Series and the Dementia Series. The Specialty Practice Series is the newest section. The issues in this series represent a collaborative effort between HIGN and specialty nursing organizations and individuals with expertise in their specialized field of practice. At the time of this writing there are only two issues in this section, Assessment of Nociceptive versus Neuropathic Pain in Older Adults, and Informal Caregivers of Older Adults at Home: Let's PREPARE!, but several more are under development or in press.

TABLE 4.1. The *Try This:®* and *How to Try This* Series

General Assessment Series:	
Try This Issue 1	SPICES: An Overall Assessment Tool for Older Adults[a]
Try This Issue 2	Katz Index of Independence in Activities of Daily Living (ADL)[a]
Try This Issue 3	Mental Status Assessment of Older Adults: The Mini-Cog[a]
Try This Issue 4	The Geriatric Depression Scale (GDS)[a]
Try This Issue 5	Predicting Pressure Ulcer Risk[a]
Try This Issue 6.1	The Pittsburgh Sleep Quality Index (PSQI)[a]
Try This Issue 6.2	The Epworth Sleepiness Scale
Try This Issue 7	Assessing Pain in Older Adults[a]
Try This Issue 8	Fall Risk Assessment[a]
Try This Issue 9	Assessing Nutrition in Older Adults[a]
Try This Issue 10	Sexuality Assessment for Older Adults[a]
Try This Issue 11.1	Urinary Incontinence Assessment in Older Adults: Part 1 – Transient Urinary Incontinence[a]
Try This Issue 11.2	Urinary Incontinence Assessment in Older Adults: Part 2 – Persistent Urinary Incontinence
Try This Issue 12	Hearing Screening in Older Adults – A Brief Hearing Loss Screener
Try This Issue 13	Confusion Assessment Method (CAM)[a]
Try This Issue 14	The Modified Caregiver Strain Index (CSI)[a]
Try This Issue 15	Elder Mistreatment Assessment[a]
Try This Issue 16.1	Beers' Criteria for Potentially Inappropriate Medication Use in the Elderly: Part I – 2002 Criteria Independent of Diagnoses or Conditions
Try This Issue 16.2	Beers' Criteria for Potentially Inappropriate Medication Use in the Elderly: Part II – 2002 Criteria Considering Diagnoses or Conditions[a]
Try This Issue 17	Alcohol Use Screening and Assessment[a]
Try This Issue 18	The Kayser-Jones Brief Oral Health Status Examination (BOHSE)
Try This Issue 19	Horowitz's Impact of Event Scale: An Assessment of Post-Traumatic Stress in Older Adults[a]
Try This Issue 20	Preventing Aspiration in Older Adults With Dysphagia[a]
Try This Issue 21	Immunizations for the Older Adult
Try This Issue 22	Assessing Family Preferences for Participation in Care of the Hospitalized Older Adults[a]
Try This Issue 23	The Lawton Instrumental Activities of Daily Living (IADL) Scale[a]
Try This Issue 24	The Hospital Admission Risk Profile (HARP)[a]

(Continued)

TABLE 4.1. The *Try This:*® and *How to Try This* Series (*Continued*)

Try This Issue 25	Confusion Assessment Method for the Intensive Care Unit (CAM-ICU)
Try This Issue 26	The Transitional Care Model (TCM): Hospital Discharge Screening Criteria for High Risk Older Adults
Try This Issue 27	General Screening Recommendations for Chronic Disease and Risk Factors in Older Adults
Specialty Practice Series:	
Try This SP1	Assessment of Nociceptive Versus Neuropathic Pain in Older Adults
Try This SP2	Informal Caregivers of Older Adults at Home: Let's PREPARE!
Dementia Series:	
Try This D1	Avoiding Restraints in Patients With Dementia[a]
Try This D2	Assessing Pain in Persons With Dementia[a]
Try This D3	Brief Evaluation of Executive Dysfunction: An Essential Refinement in the Assessment of Cognitive Impairment[a]
Try This D4	Therapeutic Activity Kits
Try This D5	Recognition of Dementia in Hospitalized Older Adults[a]
Try This D6	Wandering in the Hospitalized Older Adult[a]
Try This D7	Communication Difficulties: Assessment and Interventions[a]
Try This D8	Assessing and Managing Delirium in Persons With Dementia[a]
Try This D9	Decision Making in Older Adults With Dementia
Try This D10	Working with Families of Hospitalized Older Adults With Dementia[a]
Try This D11.1	Eating and Feeding Issues in Older Adults With Dementia: Part I: Assessment[a]
Try This D11.2	Eating and Feeding Issues in Older Adults With Dementia: Part II: Interventions

[a]Includes *How to Try This* companion video and/or print article.
Note: The *Try This:*® and *How to Try This* series are available at: http://consultgerirn.org/resources.

The Dementia Series consists of 12 issues and includes topics such as avoiding restraints, communication difficulties, and working with families of hospitalized older adults. A complete list of the issues in the Dementia Series is included in Table 4.1. Also included in the table is a notation as to which issue also includes a *How to Try This* companion.

The *Try This:*® and *How to Try This* series are publications of the Hartford Institute for Geriatric Nursing at New York University College of Nursing (HIGN). They can be found on ConsultGeriRN, the clinical resource Web site of HIGN, at http://consultgerirn.org/resources.

Primary Care

Management Guidelines for Nurse Practitioners Working With Older Adults, Second Edition

Management Guidelines for Nurse Practitioners Working With Older Adults, Second Edition, is a pocket-sized resource for all APN students and practicing nurses who provide care to older adults in ambulatory settings. It presents evidence-based information on both health promotion and disease management for older adults. The authors are all APNs who are experts both in the education of APN students and in practice related to care of older adults. It is an ideal resource for APN students' use in the clinical area.

Management Guidelines for Nurse Practitioners Working with Older Adults, Second Edition, is divided into two sections: Unit I: The Healthy Older Adult and Unit II: Managing Illness. Unit I focuses on areas related to a healthy lifestyle and health promotion, and includes exercise, nutrition, safety, sexual behavior, dental health, substance use, and immunizations. Unit II includes a chapter on more than 20 common symptoms that present in older adults, such as bowel and urinary incontinence, confusion, fatigue, involuntary weight loss, syncope, and tremor. The chapters on diagnosis and management of illness are organized by systems. Throughout these chapters, the atypical presentation of illness in older adults is emphasized. ICD-9 and CPT codes for each disease are also included. There are three appendices, Appendix A: Physiological Influences of the Aging Process, Appendix B: Laboratory Values in the Older Adult, and Appendix C: Common Tests and Their Associations with Diseases and Conditions, which provide important information that is easily found.

The authors of *Management Guidelines for Nurse Practitioners Working with Older Adults*, Second Edition, are Laurie Kennedy-Malone, PhD, GNP-BC, FAANP; Kathleen Ryan Fletcher, MSN, RN, GNP-BC, FAAN; and Lori Martin Plank, PhD, MSPH, MSN, RN, GNP-BC. The book is published by F. A. Davis in paperback format. It has also been published in Italian and Korean. A new edition entitled *Nursing Care for Older Adults: A Manual for Advanced Practice* will be published in 2012.

Primary Care Geriatrics: A Case-Based Approach, Fifth Edition

Primary Care Geriatrics: A Case-Based Approach, Fifth Edition, is a compilation of evidence-based case studies intended for use by all health care providers who care for older adults. As in the earlier editions, essential clinical information and principles related to primary care of older adults are presented within the context of the cases. Topics of the cases include the major geriatric syndromes and the diseases and disorders that are common in older adults. The content has been totally updated using an evidence-based approach whenever possible. In addition to authors who are experts in geriatric medicine, the fifth edition also includes an author who is an expert gerontological APN. This change to an interdisciplinary viewpoint is also manifested within the text. Also new in this edition are "board-type" questions in each chapter and a CD-ROM containing additional assessment tools and review questions. There is also now a consistent format for the chapters, making it easier to find information. Since its initial release, *Primary Care Geriatrics: A Case-Based Approach* has been highly regarded as an effective teaching tool for gerontological APN students. The new interdisciplinary viewpoint, CD-ROM, "board-type" questions, and other changes in the fifth edition serve to increase its value as both a teaching and learning resource, not only for gerontological APN students but for all APN students.

Primary Care Geriatrics: A Case-Based Approach, Fifth Edition, consists of 52 chapters divided into three units. Unit One: Principles and Practice presents content related to topics such as clinical implications of normal aging, geriatric assessment, clinical pharmacology, culture and ethnicity, ethics, the health care system, and a variety of health care settings. Unit Two: Geriatric Syndromes and Common Special Problems is comprised of case studies focused on the common geriatric syndromes such as falls, incontinence, delirium, constipation, pressure ulcers, and hearing and visual impairment. Also included in this unit are cases on sexual health, pain, alcoholism, and the older driver. In Unit Three: Selected Clinical Problems of the Organ Systems, the emphasis is on cases related to disorders and diseases commonly found in the older adult population.

The authors of *Primary Care Geriatrics: A Case-Based Approach*, Fifth Edition, are Richard J. Ham, MD; Philip D. Sloane, MD, MPH; Gregg A. Warshaw, MD; Marie A. Bernard, MD; and Ellen Flaherty, PhD, GNP-BC. It is published by Mosby, Inc., an affiliate of Elsevier Inc., and is available in paperback only.

Acute and Long-Term Care

Evidence-Based Geriatric Nursing Protocols for Best Practice, Third Edition

Evidence-Based Geriatric Nursing Protocols for Best Practice, Third Edition, is a comprehensive evidence-based collection of "best practices" protocols for nursing care of hospitalized older adults. Written for an audience that includes undergraduate- and graduate-level nursing students, staff nurses, nursing educators, care managers, APNs, and nursing leaders, it provides a scientific foundation for nursing care of acutely ill older adults. The editors, all renowned experts and leaders in gerontological nursing, have convened a group of experts in gerontological nursing as contributing authors. As in earlier editions, the text presents assessments and interventions for important clinical conditions and situations experienced by older adults in acute care settings. Emphasis is placed on reducing the high risk for complications that older adults face due to factors such as the physiological changes of aging, differences in presentation of illness, multiple comorbidities, and polypharmacy commonly seen in this population. The content in the third edition has been updated using the best evidence available, and contains 13 new topics that include nutrition in aging, oral health care, iatrogenesis, fluid overload, family caregiving for older adults, and cancer and the older patient. Also included in the third edition are case studies that provide an explanation of the use of the evidence and the protocol. This text is a valuable resource for all nurses, including APNs, who provide care to older adults in an acute care setting.

Evidence-Based Geriatric Nursing Protocols for Best Practice, Third Edition, consists of 29 chapters. Background content about developing clinical practice guidelines, measuring performance and improving quality, and assessment of function is discussed in the first three chapters. The remaining chapters focus on geriatric syndromes including delirium, falls, urinary incontinence, and pressure ulcers, as well as common conditions and issues in older adults such as depression, dementia, pain management, and fluid overload. In addition, there are chapters that present content related to age-related changes in health, sensory changes, iatrogenesis, nutrition, and oral hydration. Topics related to legal and ethical issues include restraint use, health care decision making, advance directives, and substance misuse.

The editors of *Evidence-Based Geriatric Nursing Protocols for Best Practice*, Third Edition, are Elizabeth Capezuti, PhD, RN, FAAN; Deanne Zwicker, MS, GNP-BC; Mathy Mezey, EdD, RN, FAAN; and Terry Fulmer, PhD, RN, FAAN. It is published by Springer Publishing Company.

Improving Hospital Care for Persons with Dementia

Improving Hospital Care for Persons with Dementia was written to highlight the issues and gaps in quality care that people with dementia experience while hospitalized, with the hope that this would ultimately lead to improved hospital care for these patients. The content is derived from the research literature, case studies, and examples of best practices. The case studies describe actual occurrences and discuss the difficulties encountered as well as the approaches used to address them. The editors, a gerontologist and a social worker with strong backgrounds in health policy, quality care advocacy, and research in the care of older adults, have assembled an interdisciplinary panel of contributing authors that includes experts in the fields of gerontological nursing, geriatric medicine, geriatric social work, public health, and dementia care. The target audience for this book ranges from direct care providers in hospitals, such as nurses, social workers, physicians, and psychologists, to hospital administrators (Silverstein & Maslow, 2006). This book is an ideal resource for the APN student in an acute care setting. The interdisciplinary nature of the book and the real-life cases provide an opportunity to gain insight into hospital care of the older adult with dementia from a variety of perspectives.

Improving Hospital Care for Persons with Dementia is divided into four parts: Part I: Background and Significance; Part II: Four Perspectives on the Hospital Experience for Persons with Dementia; Part III: Promising Approaches for Improving Care for Hospitalized Elders with Dementia; and Part IV: Strategies for Making a Difference. Part I describes the magnitude of the topic, including dissimilarities in hospital use rates for nursing home residents with Alzheimer's disease and the concept of dementia-friendly hospitals. In the second part, hospital care of the person with dementia is discussed from the perspective of assisted living providers, a geriatric social worker, emergency department personnel, and a patient with Alzheimer's disease. Part III presents four different models of hospital care for older adults with dementia, including system-wide and unit-specific approaches. The last part provides examples of successful strategies and concludes with the editors' vision for the future care of hospitalized people with dementia.

The editors of *Improving Hospital Care for Persons with Dementia* are Nina M. Silverstein, PhD, and Katie Maslow, MSW. It is published by Springer Publishing Company.

Critical Care Nursing of Older Adults: Best Practices, Third Edition

Critical Care Nursing of Older Adults: Best Practices, Third Edition, is a comprehensive evidence-based collection of "best practices" protocols for nursing care of critically ill older adults. The target audience for this book is nurses caring for older adults in intensive care units, step-down units, trauma units, and the emergency department. The content in the third edition is all-inclusive and presents evidence-based information that is essential for the delivery of comprehensive, quality nursing care to critically ill older adults. In addition to the foundations of and approaches to clinical care of critically ill older adults, also presented is content on ethical decision making, continuity of care, and the standards of practice for both gerontological and critical care nursing. The authors are all renowned experts, researchers, and leaders in gerontological nursing with a focus on acute and critical care nursing. Although written for the practicing nurse, this book provides a comprehensive evidence-based approach to nursing care of the critically ill older adult and, as such, should prove to be a useful resource for both faculty and students in acute and critical care APN programs.

Critical Care Nursing of Older Adults: Best Practices, Third Edition, consists of 26 chapters divided into four parts. Part I: The Context for Critical Care Nursing of Older Adults includes an introduction and overview of the text, the standards of practice, and chapters on the critical care environment and safety issues for older adults in intensive care. The seven chapters in Part II: Social Aspects of Critical Care Nursing of Older Adults present content related to ethical decision making, continuity of care, family responses, end-of-life care and advance directives, frailty, the chronically critically ill, and optimizing function in acute care settings. Part III: Foundations for Clinical Care of Critically Ill Older Adults focuses on physiology, pharmacotherapy, nutrition and hydration, restraint use, infections and sepsis, sleep disorders in intensive care, and pain management. The last section, Part IV: Approaches to Complex Clinical Issues in Critically Ill Older Adults, addresses common problems encountered in the critically ill older adult. They include pressure ulcers, wound healing, urinary incontinence, and delirium. Also included are chapters on substance abuse and withdrawal, heart failure, perioperative care, and acute respiratory failure and mechanical ventilation.

The authors of Critical Care Nursing of Older Adults: Best Practices, Third Edition, are Marquis D. Foreman, PhD, RN, FAAN; Koen Milisen, PhD, RN; and Terry Fulmer, PhD, RN, FAAN. It is published by Springer Publishing Company.

The Nurse Practitioner in Long-Term Care: Guidelines for Clinical Practice

The Nurse Practitioner in Long-Term Care: Guidelines for Clinical Practice is a comprehensive collection of clinical guidelines for the care of frail older adults in nursing homes. Although it was written specifically for NPs working in nursing homes, the content would also be appropriate for use by all APNs who provide care to frail older adults in other clinical settings such as primary and acute care. It is also useful for APN faculty and students in preparation for or during clinical placements in long-term care facilities. Content is derived from the best available evidence and includes general principles related to patient management in long-term care, guidelines for clinical management of common disorders, and special considerations in this population, such as wound care, podiatry, and end-of-life care. Lists of Internet resources and additional references are provided to facilitate in-depth study of the topics. The authors are adult gerontological NPs with experience in both APN education and long-term care. Long-term care residents represent a unique subset of the older adult population. There are few, if any, texts with a specific focus on the care of frail older adults and this text fills a major gap in this area. In addition, there are many frail older adults who do not reside in nursing homes but in their own homes or with their families. Therefore, this text is a valuable reference for faculty and students in all APN programs whose graduates will provide care to older adults regardless of settings.

The Nurse Practitioner in Long-Term Care: Guidelines for Clinical Practice comprises 23 chapters divided into three sections: Section I: General Principles; Section II: Management Guidelines for Common Disorders; and Section III: Special Considerations. The first section includes chapters on general patient management, health promotion and disease prevention, and legal and ethical issues. The common disorders presented in Section II are organized by systems and are all-inclusive. The chapters in this section include the epidemiology, assessment, diagnostic workup, and both pharmacological and nonpharmacological management for each disorder. Special considerations discussed in the third section are wound care, nutrition, rehabilitation in a skilled nursing facility, podiatry, pain management, and end-of-life care.

The authors of *The Nurse Practitioner in Long-Term Care: Guidelines for Clinical Practice* are Barbara White, DrPH, APRN, BC, and Deborah Truax, MS, APRN, BC. It is published by Jones and Bartlett Publishers.

SELECTED GERIATRIC JOURNALS

Geriatric Nursing

Geriatric Nursing is a comprehensive, monthly, peer-reviewed journal targeted to all nurses who provide care to older adults. It is a "cutting edge" journal in geriatrics with articles that present the latest developments, as well as practical advice, on clinical topics across the continuum of care. There are monthly columns that discuss current issues related to pharmacology, legal issues, acute care, and assisted living. It is the official journal of the Gerontological Advanced Practice Nurses Association (GAPNA), the National Gerontological Nurses Association (NGNA), and the American Assisted Living Nurses Association. Both GAPNA and NGNA have sections devoted to content written by their members. Although the intended audience for *Geriatric Nursing* is all nurses, the overall content and presentation is at the advanced practice level making it an indispensable resource for the integration of gerontological content into APN programs.

Geriatric Nursing is included as a membership benefit for the above organizations, in both print and online versions. It is also available in print by individual subscription. Academic institutions can subscribe to it as an ejournal, making it readily and freely available to students and faculty. It is indexed in Medline, ISI, and CINAHL. *Geriatric Nursing* is an Elsevier publication and information about the journal can be found at http://www.gnjournal.com/home.

Journal of Gerontological Nursing

Published by Slack, Incorporated, the *Journal of Gerontological Nursing* is a monthly, peer-reviewed journal for nurses who provide care to older adults in a variety of settings. Each issue contains feature articles on topics that are clinically relevant to the care of older adults and includes one article that offers continuing nursing education contact hours. There are sections that present content on a rotating variety of topics that include pharmacology, dementia, legal issues, public policy, and clinical concepts. Regular departments provide monthly updates on new products, Foundation activities, and recent research findings related to the care of older adults. Although this journal is primarily targeted to basic registered nurses, it does feature content that is relevant to APN students, such as the evidence-based guideline on acute confusion and delirium in the November 2009 issue and the clinical concepts article on risks for an older patient in the emergency department in the December 2009 issue.

The *Journal of Gerontological Nursing* is available through individual and institutional subscriptions. Individual subscribers will benefit from a new Online Advanced Release, which allows them to read articles before they appear in the print issue. Information about the journal can be found at http://www.jognonline.com/default.asp.

Journal of the American Geriatrics Society

The *Journal of the American Geriatrics Society* is a monthly, peer-reviewed interdisciplinary journal with a primary focus on clinical care of older adults. Content is comprehensive in scope and includes topics that have an immediate-, intermediate-, or long-range potential benefit to practice. It is composed of a number of sections, such as Clinical Investigations, Drugs and Pharmacology, Ethics, Nursing, Public Policy, and Models of Geriatric Care, which appear on a rotating basis in different issues of the journal. Examples of some of the topics addressed in the journal include biological aspects of aging, psychosocial issues, legal and ethical issues, care of the older adult in different care settings, geriatric assessment, prevention, palliative care, complementary and alternative medicine, nursing, geriatric syndromes, geriatric psychiatry, and diseases and disorders common in older adults. The comprehensive interdisciplinary nature of this journal makes it an ideal resource for faculty and students in all APN programs.

The *Journal of the American Geriatrics Society* is included as a membership benefit in the American Geriatrics Society. It is also available as institutional and individual subscriptions for print and online versions. It is published by Wiley-Blackwell and information about the journal may be found at http://www.wiley.com/bw/journal.asp?ref=0002861 4&site=1.

Annals of Long-Term Care: Clinical Care and Aging

Another journal from the American Geriatrics Society is *Annals of Long-Term Care: Clinical Care and Aging*. It is a monthly, peer-reviewed, clinical journal that addresses the care of older adults in long-term care settings and is targeted to all members of the health care team: nurse practitioners, attending physicians, consultant pharmacists, geriatric psychiatrists, directors of nursing, and medical directors. Content consists of articles and columns related to the assorted diagnoses and health problems commonly seen in older adults in long-term care settings. Each issue also includes one of the *Try This:®* Series from the Hartford Institute for Geriatric Nursing. Periodically, the journal produces supplemental issues and special projects monographs, which are available to subscribers. This journal is designed for the busy practitioner with articles that are focused and concise. It is a good resource for APN students during clinical experiences in long-term care facilities. In addition, print and online subscriptions are offered at no cost to all health care professionals, including both practicing and student APNs, making it an ideal choice for all APN students who care for older adults.

The *Annals of Long-Term Care: Clinical Care and Aging* is a publication of HMP Communications. More information about the journal and the subscription application can be found at http://www.annalsoflongtermcare. com/.

SUMMARY

In keeping with the purpose of this text, to facilitate the integration of gerontological content into curricula by faculty in nongerontological APN programs, this chapter presented an annotated list of print media resources of gerontological content created for use by faculty in nongerontological APN programs. The resources were selected from the work of multiple disciplines and ranged in content from health promotion to long-term care. Each of the resources was described with regard to its relevance to APN education. This chapter and the one that follows, which addresses gerontological/geriatric Internet resources, provide APN faculty with a comprehensive list of initial resources.

REFERENCES

Auerhahn, C., Capezuti, E., Flaherty, E., & Resnick, B. (Eds.). (2007). *Geriatric nursing review syllabus: A core curriculum in advanced practice geriatric nursing* (2nd ed.). New York: American Geriatrics Society.

Capezuti, E., Zwicker, D., Mezey, M., & Fulmer, T. (Eds.). (2008). *Evidence-based geriatric nursing protocols for best practice* (3rd ed.). New York: Springer Publishing Company.

Foreman, M. D., Milisen, K., & Fulmer, T. (Eds.). (2009). *Critical care nursing of older adults: Best practices* (3rd ed.). New York: Springer Publishing Company.

Gallo, J. J., Bogner, H. R., Fulmer, T., & Paveza, G. J. (Eds.). (2006). *Handbook of geriatric assessment* (4th ed.). Boston: Jones and Bartlett Publishers.

Haber, D. (2010). *Health promotion and aging: Practical applications for health professionals* (5th ed.). New York: Springer Publishing Company.

Halter, J. B., Ouslander, J. G., Tinetti, M. E., Studenski, S., High, K. P., & Asthana, S. (Eds.). (2009). *Hazzard's geriatric medicine & gerontology* (6th ed.). New York: The McGraw-Hill Companies.

Ham, R. J., Sloane, P. D., Warshaw, G. A., Bernard, M. A., & Flaherty, E. (2007). *Primary care geriatrics: A case-based approach* (5th ed.). St. Louis: Mosby, Inc., an affiliate of Elsevier Inc.

Hartford Institute for Geriatric Nursing (HIGN). (2009). *Try This:®* and *How to Try This* series. New York: Author.

Kane, R., Ouslander, J., Abrass, I., & Resnick, B. (2008). *Essentials of clinical geriatrics* (6th ed.). New York: McGraw-Hill Professional.

Kennedy-Malone, L., Fletcher, K. R., & Plank, L. M. (2004). *Management guidelines for nurse practitioners working with older adults* (2nd ed.). Philadelphia: F. A. Davis.

Miller, C. A. (2009). *Nursing for wellness in older adults* (5th ed.). Philadelphia: Wolters Kluwer Health/Lippincott Williams & Wilkins.

Nolan, M. R. (2009). Clinical concepts: Older patients in the emergency department: What are the risks? *Journal of Gerontological Nursing, 35*(12), 14–18.

Reuben, D. B., Herr, K. A., Pacala, J. T., Pollock, B. G., Potter, J. F., & Semla, T. P. (2009). *Geriatrics at your fingertips*™ (11th ed.). New York: American Geriatrics Society.

Sendlebach, S., Guthrie, P. F., & Schoenfelder, D. P. (2009). Evidence-based guideline: Acute confusion/delirium, identification, assessment, treatment, and prevention. *Journal of Gerontological Nursing, 35*(11), 11–18.

Silverstein, N. M., & Maslow, K. (Eds.). (2006). *Improving hospital care for persons with dementia.* New York: Springer Publishing Company.

White, B., & Truax, D. (2007). *The nurse practitioner in long-term care: Guidelines for clinical practice.* Boston: Jones and Bartlett Publishers.

CHAPTER 5

Internet Resources for Enhancing Gerontological Content in Advanced Practice Nursing Curriculum

Laurie Kennedy-Malone

As nursing faculty, we are faced now with the task of enhancing the APN curriculum to address the needs of our rapidly aging, diverse population. Given the demands on faculty's time, however, and the need to incorporate existing national standards and curriculum guidelines, it can be challenging, even daunting, to meet requirements for curricular expansion. This chapter first describes select geriatric- and gerontology-focused Web-based sites. These online clearinghouses provide access to a wide range of E-learning materials available for faculty to integrate geriatric content into the curriculum. Second, additional portals to E-learning materials that contain learning objects pertinent to health care, nursing, and/or medical education are described. Select academic and organizational Web sites that contain geriatric and gerontological educational resources are highlighted. Finally, strategies to identify and include gerontological learning objects and enhancing overall E-learning opportunities for students are presented.

INTEGRATING GERONTOLOGICAL E-LEARNING MATERIALS INTO THE APN CURRICULM

There is a trend now in health care education to incorporate a blended learning approach as a means of integrating gerontological content in the academic curricula of nongeriatric specialty programs (Ruiz, Mintzer, &

Leipzig, 2006). For years faculty have complemented teacher-delivered lectures with videos and slide presentations depicting clinical scenarios. According to Ruiz, Mintzer, and Issenberg (2006), the use of digital learning objects is easing the faculty burden of "meeting challenges of competing priorities" (p. 599), as is the case of APN faculty charged with adding gerontological content to an already burgeoning curriculum. Learning objects are defined "as any entity, digital or nondigital, which can be used, re-used or referenced during technology supported learning. Examples of technology-supported learning include computer-based training systems, interactive learning environments, intelligent computer-aided instruction systems, distance learning systems, and collaborative learning environments" (Wiley, 2000, pp. 4–5). With the advent of learning management systems, APN faculty now have the ability to direct students to specific digital learning objects such as videos, Web-based tutorials, computer-assisted simulations, and recorded heart and lungs sound, to name a few (Ruiz, van Zuilen, Kai, & Mintzer, 2005). The use of E-learning materials in geriatric education has numerous advantages for faculty lacking adequate expertise in gerontological nursing. Educational resources developed by gerontological experts are readily available for faculty to include in the courses, many of which are designed to be reusable in diverse educational contexts (Ruiz, Mintzer, & Issenberg, 2006). Throughout this book, Web-based and multimedia gerontological resources have been recommended for faculty to consider, including in APN curriculum, as one means of infusing more gerontological content into a competency-based curriculum.

Navigating Through Web-Based Geriatric Educational Resources

When an extensive search of four common search engines—Yahoo, Google, AltaVista, and MedHunt—using the term "geriatric education" was performed, over 170,000 sites were identified (Hirth & Hajjar, 2004). With the growing number of geriatric education-specific Web sites available, APN faculty have access to a wide array of E-learning materials that can be incorporated into Web-based courses and face-to-face, teacher-led presentations. Navigating through the vast array of geriatric educational materials can be overwhelming to educators, especially those without expertise in geriatrics and gerontological nursing. The need to personally determine the credibility of the online materials now has been greatly reduced with the introduction of online clearinghouses of information that often provide peer-reviews of the submitted learning objects. APN faculty will benefit greatly from familiarizing themselves with online digital libraries, known as repositories, to search for electronic gerontological educational resources. Some of the popular geriatric and health care repositories as well as one referatory site are described in the upcoming section. Geriatric educational material is also highlighted on academic centers' Web sites and sites of professional organizations.

The Portal of Geriatric Online Education (POGOe)

The Portal of Geriatric Online Education (POGOe), a free public repository of emerging geriatric educational materials developed by faculty in the field of geriatric medicine and gerontology, is available to faculty interested in enhancing gerontological content in NP and CNS curriculum. POGOe, funded by the Donald W. Reynolds Foundation, was originally developed as a means for recipients of funding from the foundation to disseminate educational materials. POGOe is managed by the Mount Sinai School of Medicine Department of Geriatrics and Adult Development, and is a partnership between Mount Sinai and Vanderbilt University School of Medicine (POGOe, 2009). This clearinghouse that can be accessed at www.pogoe.org contains E-learning materials such as case-based discussions, virtual patients, simulations, and audio conferences. Links to various Web-based resources for geriatric medical information are also available (Ruiz, Teasdale, Hajjar, Shaughnessy, & Mintzer, 2007). To access the materials on POGOe, visitors are required to register their identifying information and log in each time they access the site. Very helpful features found on POGOe are the reviews of products available for download and/or purchase. By previewing the products available, faculty can read descriptions of the product and the educational objectives intended for use with the product in order to determine the applicability of the materials to the curriculum. E-learning resources that have been peer-reviewed will be noted as part of the product description. It is highly recommended that faculty sign up to receive the monthly email newsletter (e-newsletter) from POGOe. Featured in the newsletter are announcements to site updates and upcoming events in geriatric medical and gerontology education. New products added to POGOe by faculty are described and links are added to direct the viewer to seek additional information. New materials developed by faculty may be submitted to POGOe for inclusion in the repository. The *Journal of the American Geriatrics Society* publishes reviews of new materials submitted to POGOe (POGOe Newsletter, April 2009).

GeriatricWeb

Known as the "Geriatric Resources for Healthcare Professionals," GeriatricWeb, which can be found at http://geriatricweb.sc.edu/, is a repository of gerontological and health care–related information. The National Library of Medicine, the University of South Carolina School of Medicine, and the Division of Geriatrics at Palmetto Health Care Richland Hospital are cosponsors of this site. Information presented on this Web site is continuously updated to reflect current clinical management practices, standardized assessment tools, educational resources, practice guidelines, and current clinical trials. Hot topics in geriatric medicine are highlighted and links to additional geriatric Web sites are included on the home page. Available learning objects include video clips and images that can be retrieved for presentations and/or inclusion on course management sites. Of benefit to faculty and students is the ability to directly download information to a PDA or similar handheld device. Professional reviews of the material on GeriatricWeb are available for faculty to quickly scan the information that will be found on the links to other sites that will aid in the selection of E-learning materials.

ConsultGeriRN.org

When searching information specific to gerontological nursing, Consult-GeriRN.org is an excellent Web-based resource for APN faculty to visit regularly. It provides up-to-date geriatric evidenced-based protocols for managing common geriatric syndromes. Information formerly housed on GeroNurseOnline.org can be found at this site now at http://consultgerirn. org/. Funded in part by a grant from The Atlantic Philanthropies (USA) Inc. and The John A. Hartford Foundation, ConsultGeriRN.org provides faculty and students access to an extensive list of geriatric resources, including links to aging associations and societies, educational resources, gerontological certification information, and recommended books and journals, as well as scope and standards of practice.

A distinct feature that APN faculty will find very beneficial on this site is The Geriatrics and the Advanced Practice Curriculum: A Series of Web-Based Interactive Case Studies. These case studies were developed as a way for faculty to integrate geriatric content into nongerontological APN programs. Following a tutorial format, the students become active participants in managing the care of the older adult in this problem-based learning activity (Thornlow, Auerhahn, & Stanley, 2006). Five clinical cases, with content that is cross-referenced to the *Nurse Practitioner and Clinical Nurse Specialist Competencies for Older Adult Care* (American Association of Colleges of Nursing [AACN], 2004), are available for students to enter responses to questions about the patients. Immediate feedback is provided to the students after their responses are submitted. Direct links to the cases can be added to the course management system the university uses for Web-based courses. These cases can be retrieved at the following site: http://hartfordign.org/continuing_ed/case_studies/

Direct access to the *Try This:®* and *How to Try This* series is located when clicking the clinical resources/tools button. Available for direct download are the assessment tools, articles pertaining to the tools, and short video clips describing the use of the tools in clinical practice. The information provided on both the *Try This:®* and *How to Try This* may be downloaded and printed for educational use. APN faculty may consider assigning the various assessment tools as part of ongoing clinical assignments when students are working with older adults. Providing the link to the accompanying video on your course management site or embedded in lecture presentation can be very valuable for students beginning to build their clinical assessment skills with older adults.

APN faculty preparing presentations on aging and gerontological nursing may retrieve images from the Geriatric Picture link located on this site. Select information is also available in Spanish. Faculty are encouraged to sign up for the e-newsletter to receive notices of new information uploaded to the Web site.

GEC National Online Directory

Through a portal hosted by the Central Plains Geriatric Education Center at the University of Kansas Medical Center, faculty can access materials that have been developed by Geriatric Education Centers (GEC) throughout the United States. GEC Clearinghouse accessed at http://coa.kumc.edu/gecresource/ has a convenient feature in the Quick Search ability. Faculty can locate information by title, keyword, product type, media type, and audience, as well as by organizations that have developed a specific product. Educational resources are listed by the GEC that designed the material, which are either free for download or require a fee for purchase.

Clinical Toolbox for Geriatric Care

The Clinical Toolbox for Geriatric Care was developed by the Society of Hospital Medicine's Geriatric Task Force. The toolbox, which can be accessed at http://www.hospitalmedicine.org/geriresource/toolbox/howto. htm, contains clinical information for geriatric specialists who work across a variety of practice sites; general geriatric resources for inpatient elder care are highlighted, however. The viewer can select one of the categories listed and find a brief description of the strengths, weaknesses, and context for use of the item. Of value to all APNs caring for older adults are the various mental status, functional assessment, and pain assessment tools. Included on the Web site are clinical practice guidelines, as well as useful information pertaining to hospitalization and discharge care. The full resource is discussed and interpretive guides are available in downloadable files.

MedEdPORTAL

While not a site specific to geriatric education, APN faculty will find MedEdPORTAL of value when searching for multimedia resources available for download or direct access. MedEdPORTAL is a service provided by the Association of American Medical Colleges (AAMC) in partnership with the American Dental Education Association (ADEA). All users will be required to register to use the resources on MedEdPORTAL and log in each time the site is accessed; the service, however, is free for participants. This online peer-reviewed publication service facilitates the exchange of a variety of E-learning resources such as simulations, virtual patients, videos, and assessment tools. When you select a resource to view, a detailed abstract is presented that provides information about the author of the learning object, means to access the material such as direct download, or a direction to an external Web site with details about when the content was last updated. To keep abreast of new information added to the site, faculty are encouraged to sign up for the monthly newsletter. MedEdPORTAL can be found at www.aamc.org/mededportal.

MERLOT

The Multimedia Educational Resource for Learning and Online Teaching, known as MERLOT, is a "referatory" of a wide range of educational resources. MERLOT is located at www.merlot.org. To access information pertaining to older adults, APN faculty may select a number of key phrases such as geriatrics or aging to access materials. The information found after searching the topic is further delineated by material type such as game, tutorial, or lecture/presentation. Faculty will also have access to any peer review comments about the materials and how others have used the learning object (Sewell, 2006). One can also browse the discipline community of Health Science for additional information. A more extensive search of other learning object repositories can be accessed if one selects "federated search" when clicking the search button.

Access to MERLOT is free; however, if one wishes to become a member, registration is required to post learning objects to the site as well as add resources to their personal collection. Members of MERLOT will receive the MERLOT Grapevine Newsletter via email. Subscribers to MERLOT also have access to the *Journal of Learning and Online Teaching (JOLT)*, which is a peer-reviewed, online, quarterly publication dedicated to the scholarly use of multimedia resources in education. A new feature in MERLOT is the ability to access MERLOT Mobile Search using your mobile phone. This application can be downloaded at http://mobile.merlot.org

Academic Web-Based Gerontological Educational Resources

Excellent sources for up-to-date educational resources can be found on geriatric medicine, nursing, social work, and other allied health-profession programs' academic Web sites. Many academic programs that supplement the traditional educational process with online resources have made available geriatric E-learning materials, often developed as part of a grant funded by foundations with the purpose of widely disseminating the educational products (Hirth & Hajjar, 2004). Most often, the learning objects available on these Web sites can be accessed directly while searching the geriatric repositories such as POGOe and GeriatricWeb. Additionally, if a university is a funded Geriatric Education Center (GEC), then materials can also be accessed at the GEC Clearinghouse Web site. A select listing of academic–based gerontological Web sites with a brief description of information that can be found on these sites is described in Table 5.1.

Gerontological Organization Web-Based Resources

Gerontological Nursing Organizations

When seeking up-to-date information on geriatric clinical practice guidelines and educational standards, it is most beneficial to periodically visit

TABLE 5.1. Select Academic Web-Based Gerontological Educational Resources

Academic Center	Description of Geriatric Web-Based Resources
The University of Iowa Geriatric Education	
GeriaSims http://www.healthcare.uiowa.edu/igec/ resources-educators-professionals/ geriasims/Default.asp	GeriaSims are interactive "virtual patient" simulations on issues encountered in the care of older patients. Topics include falls, polypharmacy, dementia, delirium, ischemic stroke, and failure to thrive.
GeriaFlix & GeriaTrax http://www.healthcare.uiowa.edu/igec/ resources-educators-professionals/ presentations/Default.asp	GeriaFlix & GeriaTrax are multi-disciplinary presentations on topics in clinical geriatrics presented in a streaming digital video and/or audio format with synchronized slides
Virginia Commonwealth University	
Geriatric Pharmacotherapy Cases http://www.virginiageriatrics.org/ casestudies/pharmacotherapy/ index.html	Interactive geriatric pharmacotherapy cases
Geriatric Clinical Management Cases http://www.virginiageriatrics.org/ casestudies/pulmoGImusc/index.htm	Interactive case studies that allow students to follow patients with comorbidities of acute and chronic conditions
University of Florida Geriatrics Education Center http://medinfo.ufl.edu/~gec/coa3/ coa3intro.html	A series of six audiocassette modules, Caring for the Older Adult III, are interactive educational programs designed for health professionals across the continuum of care settings for older adults.
The Donald W. Reynolds Department of Geriatric Medicine at the University of Oklahoma http://www.oumedicine. com/body.cfm?id=3588	Online resources/interactive case studies on topics such as geriatric rheumatology, pressure ulcers, and oral health
The University of California San Francisco Academic Geriatric Resource Center Online curriculum http://ucsfagrc.org/curriculum_home.html	A series of core and supplemental modules designed to be used by multiple disciplines seeking to increase knowledge on normal aging.

the Web sites of the prominent geriatric and gerontological organizations and foundations. Gerontological Advanced Practice Nursing Association (GAPNA), formally known as the National Conference of Gerontological Nurse Practitioners (NCGNP), can be accessed at www.gapna.org. Available are online continuing education opportunities, position statements, and the GAPNA newsletter, which contains informative articles on the practice, research, and education of advanced practice gerontological nursing. The Web site of the National Gerontological Nursing Association (NGNA) found at www.ngna.org provides excellent links to geriatric resources, clinical fast facts, and position statements.

Geriatric Medical Organizations

A great resource that can be accessed from the Web site of the American Geriatrics Society (AGS) is the downloadable version of *Geriatrics at Your Fingertips.* Students can access this publication that can be installed on a handheld device if they register as an online student and nonvoting member of the AGS. Other valuable resources found on the AGS Web site at www.americangeriatrics.org include AGS practice guidelines, clinical practice tools, and patient education materials. In seeking information specific to medical management of older adults in long-term care, it is recommended that the Web site for the American Medical Directors Association (AMDA) is frequented for information on clinical practice guidelines. AMDA can be accessed at www.amda. com. Faculty teaching in psychiatric APN programs may find valuable clinical information on the care of the older adult with mental health issues on the Web page for American Association for Geriatric Psychiatry found at http://www. aagpgpa.org/.

Interdisciplinary Gerontological Organizations and Associations

The Association of Gerontology in Higher Education (AGHE) is a national organization devoted to gerontological education. Nursing faculty can access a wide range of educational resources by visiting http://www.aghe.org/. The Gerontological Society of America (GSA) is an organization founded to promote the scientific study of aging, and is composed of researchers, practitioners, educators, and others with an interest in gerontology. Information about GSA can be found at www.geron.org. Faculty who teach information on public policy would benefit from visiting the Web site of the National Academy on an Aging Society at http://www.agingsociety.org and subscribing to the free *Public Policy and Aging* e-newsletter.

Additional information on healthy aging and age-related health care, public policy for the aging, caregiving and other related areas can be found on the Web sites for the following: National Council on Aging (www.ncoa.org), The American Society on Aging (www.asaging.org), and the American Association of Retired Persons (AARP) (www.aarp.org).

STRATEGIES FOR INTEGRATING GERIATRIC E-LEARNING MATERIALS INTO APN CURRICULUM

Throughout this book, the recommendation for integrating gerontological content into the APN curriculum has been directed toward competency-based education. Numerous examples of geriatric Web-based resources have been identified for faculty to incorporate in graduate-level, core, support, and specialty APN courses. Faculty are encouraged to adapt blended learning methodologies to include gerontological content into the APN curriculum (Ruiz et al., 2005). They should identify geriatric E-learning materials that students can complete independently to supplement curricular content already contained in the academic programs and, at the same time, can be linked directly to advanced practice "gero-rich" nursing curriculum (Thornlow et al., 2006).

Using the academic learning management system subscribed to by their university, faculty can include links to the specific learning objects (videos and online modules), thereby creating a course-specific "repository" of geriatric educational materials that students can access asynchronously and repeatedly as necessary (Ruiz, Kai, Smith, Granville, Williams, Mintzer, & Roos, 2002). Many of the commercial sites now have the option of adding Web-based portfolios for students to record their progress in attaining competency throughout the duration of their academic program. APN students in nongerontological programs can be encouraged to record, in a Web-based portfolio, their gerontological clinical experiences and the experiential learning activities in which they have participated throughout the program, such as geriatric-focused objective structured clinical examinations (Dannefer & Henson, 2007; Supiano, Fantone, & Grum, 2002).

The addition of E-learning gerontological resources to complement the APN curriculum will need to be evaluated. Faculty should consider formative evaluation of each course from the following standpoints: attainment of learner knowledge, demonstration of competency, and student satisfaction with the blended-learning format (Ruiz et al., 2006), The outcomes of enhanced gerontological curriculum should be measured by job placement and employer satisfaction of APN with the ability to safely manage the care of older adults.

SUMMARY

Infusing gerontological content across the APN curriculum is now a necessity for nursing faculty. The use of Internet-based resources are now commonplace in medical educational programs, meeting the challenge of integrating gerontological content into nongeriatric specialty curriculum (Hajjar, Ruiz, Teasdale, & Mintzer, 2007). APN faculty are encouraged to adopt the same blended-learning approach used by medicine whereby geriatric learning objects complement existing graduate nursing-level curricula and at the same time allow for attainment of specific competencies identified in the *Nurse Practitioner and Clinical Nurse Specialist Competencies for Older Adult Care* (AACN, 2004). E-learning material should include resources for student self-paced learning and remediation as needed. For example, providing the students with access to Web-based clinical case studies that provide instant feedback can be beneficial for students preparing not only for a specific course, but later in preparation for national certification examinations that include content on managing the care of older adults.

This chapter has provided a brief overview of some of the more well-known Web-based repositories for gerontological and geriatric E-learning material. It is highly recommended that APN faculty peruse the online clearinghouses of information to first search for learning objects to include not only in their Web-based courses, but to enhance face-to-face lecture presentations with images and video clips found on the Web site. By subscribing to the repository e-newsletter, faculty can be alerted to new acquisitions on the portal. Once familiar with the select learning objects, faculty are encouraged to post their individual reviews on how the items are used to enhance the curriculum. Finally, faculty who have developed E-learning objects are encouraged to submit their materials for peer review.

REFERENCES

American Association of Colleges of Nursing (AACN). (2004). *Nurse practitioner and clinical nurse specialist competencies for older adult care*. Washington, DC: Author.

American Association for Geriatric Psychiatry [online]. Retrieved October 12, 2009, from http://www.aagpgpa.org/

American Association of Retired Persons (AARP) [online]. Retrieved October 12, 2009, from www.aarp.org

American Geriatrics Society (AGS). [online]. Retrieved October 12, 2009, from www.americangeriatrics.org

American Medical Directors Association (AMDA) [online]. Retrieved October 12, 2009, from www.amda.com

American Society on Aging (ASA) [online]. Retrieved October 11, 2009, from www.asaging.org

Association of Gerontology in Higher Education (AGHE) [online]. Retrieved October 12, 2009, from www.aghe.org

Clinical Toolbox for Geriatric Care [online]. Retrieved October 12, 2009, from http://www.hospitalmedicine.org/geriresource/toolbox/howto.htm

Dannefer, E. F., & Henson, L. C. (2007). The portfolio approach to a competency-based assessment at the Cleveland Clinic Lerner College of Medicine. *Academic Medicine: Journal of the American Medical Colleges*, 82(5), 493–502.

Gerontological Advanced Practice Nurses Association (GAPNA) [online]. Retrieved October 12, 2009, from https://www.gapna.org/

Gerontological Educational Centers (GEC) National Online Directory [online]. Retrieved June 13, 2009, from http://coa.kumc.edu/gecresource/

Gerontological Society of America (GSA) [online]. Retrieved October 12, 2009, from www.geron.org

GeriatricWeb [online]. Retrieved May 23, 2009, from http://geriatricweb.sc.edu/about.cfm.

Hajjar, I. M., Ruiz, J. G., Teasdale, T. A., & Mintzer, M. J. (2007). The use of the Internet in geriatrics education: Results of a national survey of medical geriatrics academic programs. *Gerontology & Geriatrics Education*, 27(4), 85–95.

Hartford Institute for Geriatric Nursing. (2009). *ConsultGeriRN.org* [online]. Retrieved June 13, 2009, from http://consultgerirn.org/

Hirth, V. A., & Hajjar, I. (2004). Web-based framework for improving geriatric education. *Gerontology & Geriatrics Education*, 25(2), 43–55.

MedEdPORTAL [online]. Retrieved October 12, 2009, from www.aamc.org/mededportal

Multimedia Educational Resource for Learning and Online Teaching: MERLOT [online]. Retrieved July 20, 2009, from www.merlot.org

National Academy on an Aging Society [online]. Retrieved October 12, 2009, from http://www.agingsociety.org

National Council on Aging [online]. Retrieved October 12, 2009, from www. ncoa.org

National Gerontological Nurses Association (NGNA) [online]. Retrieved October 10, 2009, from www.ngna.org

POGOe. Portal of Online Geriatrics Education [online]. Retrieved May 22, 2009, from www.pogoe.org

Ruiz, J., Kai, T., Smith, M., Granville, L., Williams, C., Mintzer, M., & Roos, B. A. (2002). *GeriU*, the Online Geriatrics University (www.geriu.org): Enhancing geriatrics education through web-based learning. *Journal of the American Geriatrics Society, 50*, S72.

Ruiz, J., van Zuilen, M., Kai, T., & Mintzer, M. J. (2005). Blended learning and geriatrics education. In M. O. Thirunarayanan & Aixa Perez-Prado (Eds.), *Integrating technology in higher education* (pp. 177–195). Lanham, MD: University Press of America.

Ruiz, J. G., Mintzer, M. J., & Issenberg, S. B. (2006). Learning objects in medical education. *Medical Teacher, 28*(7), 599–605.

Ruiz, J., Mintzer, M. J., & Leipzig, R. M. (2006). The impact of E-learning on medical education. *Academic Medicine: Journal of the American Medical Colleges, 81*(3), 207–212.

Ruiz, J. G., Teasdale, T. A., Hajjar, I., Shaughnessy, M., & Mintzer, M. J. (2007). The consortium of e-learning in geriatrics instruction. *Journal of the American Geriatrics Society, 55*(3), 458–463.

Sewell, J. (2006). Best practices in teaching design: Using online learning resources in MERLOT. *CIN: Computers, Informatics, Nursing, 24*(3), 129–131.

Supiano, M. A., Fantone, J. C., & Grum, C. (2002). A web-based geriatrics portfolio to document medical students' learning outcomes. *Academic Medicine: Journal of the American Medical Colleges, 77*(9), 937–938.

Thornlow, D. K., Auerhahn, C., & Stanley, J. (2006). A necessity not a luxury: Preparing advanced practice nurses to care for older adults. *Journal of Professional Nursing, 22*(2), 116–122.

Wiley, D. A. (2000). Connecting learning objects to instructional design theory: A definition, a metaphor, and a taxonomy. In D. A. Wiley (Ed.), *The instructional use of learning objects: Online version*. Retrieved June 27, 2009, from the World Wide Web: http://reusability.org/read/chapters/wiley.doc

Methodology for
Integration of
Gerontological Content
Into Advanced Practice
Nursing Curriculum

A Competency-Based Framework for the Integration of Gerontological Content Into Nongerontological Advanced Practice Nursing Programs

Carolyn Auerhahn

Beginning in the 1970s, the competency-based education movement has gained momentum over the last two decades, and in the health professions, it is gaining recognition as the "gold standard" (APRN Consensus Work Group and National Council of State Boards of Nursing [APRN & NCSBN], 2008; Institute of Medicine [IOM], 2003; Mazurat & Schönwetter, 2008–2009; NTF, 2008). In its publication, *Health Professions Education: A Bridge to Quality,* IOM (2003) recommends that there should be one set of core competencies across the health professions, and that licensure and certification should be competency based. In the Consensus Document, the foundation for each of the four components of the LACE model—Licensure, Accreditation, Certification and Education—are competencies (APRN & NCSBN, 2008). Competencies provide the basis for NP (National Organization of Nurse Practitioner Faculties [NONPF], 2006) and CNS (National Association of Clinical Nurse Specialists [NACNS], 2004) educational programs and the graduates of these programs are expected to be able to practice according to these competencies. Within this context, and in keeping with the stated purpose of this text, "to facilitate the integration of gerontological content into curricula by faculty in nongerontological APN programs," this chapter will impart a competency-based framework designed to achieve this purpose.

The chapter is divided into two sections. The first will discuss the *Nurse Practitioner and Clinical Nurse Specialist Competencies for Older Adult Care* (AACN, 2004) with an emphasis on its relationship to other APN competency documents. The second section will explain the competency-based framework with an emphasis on the process involved. It will also describe a tool developed by the authors to facilitate the task of integrating gerontological content into nongerontological APN curricula. The process and use of the tool is modeled in Chapters 7, 8, and 9, which will provide guidance for the integration of the gerontological content into graduate nursing core, APN core, and specialty courses, respectively.

AACN/HARTFORD: *NURSE PRACTITIONER AND CLINICAL NURSE SPECIALIST COMPETENCIES FOR OLDER ADULT CARE*

The *Nurse Practitioner and Clinical Nurse Specialist Competencies for Older Adult Care* (AACN/JAHF Competencies) is the product of an initiative led by AACN and funded by the John A. Hartford Foundation (JAHF). The purpose of this initiative was to develop of a set of gerontological competencies for all APNs who provide care to older adults and was a direct response to the projected growth of the population over 65 (AACN, 2004).

This section of the chapter includes a summary of the impetus for the initiative, an overview of the process used in the development of the AACN/JAHF Competencies, the relationship of this document to other APN competency documents, and a description of the competencies contained in this document. Also included is an explanation of the design of the AACN/JAHF Competencies as a tool for the integration of gerontological content into nongerontological APN programs. A copy of the complete document is available from AACN at http://www.aacn.nche.edu/Education/pdf/APNCompetencies.pdf.

Impetus for the Initiative

As the 21st century dawned, it became evident that despite numerous attempts by schools of nursing and professional nursing organizations to prepare a nursing workforce of sufficient quality and size to care for the growing population of older adults, more were needed. Although APNs were being educated to provide care for an increasingly diverse population and across multiple specialties, the number of APNs with the necessary knowledge and skills to care for older adults was simply not adequate to meet the increasing health care demands of this growing population. An initiative of sufficient magnitude that would motivate schools of nursing and health care systems to make the necessary changes to increase their ability to produce APNs with this knowledge and skills was needed (AACN, 2004).

During this same time period, competency development for primary care and specialty practice was in progress by the National Organization of Nurse Practitioner Faculties (NONPF) and the National Association of Clinical Nurse Specialists (NACNS). There was also an ongoing national effort, funded by the Department of Health and Human Services, Health Resources and Services Administration, Bureau of Health Professions, Division of Nursing (henceforth to be called Division of Nursing) and JAHF, to provide support for care of the older adult in graduate nursing education and practice. Within this context, and because NPs and CNSs in a variety of specialties and settings provide care for a high percentage of older adults, an initiative focused on the development of competencies for care of older adults by NPs and CNSs in nongerontological specialties was judged to be an appropriate approach to the problem (AACN, 2004).

Process Used in the Development of the AACN/JAHF Competencies

A consensus-building process was used to develop and validate the AACN/JAHF Competencies. An Expert Panel, consisting of NP and CNS educators and practitioners across specialties, and an independent Validation Panel, consisting of representatives of NP, CNS, and nursing-related organizations, with the points of view of both education and practice, were selected. The members of the Expert Panel were charged with the creation of a core set of competencies related to care of older adults for both NPs and CNSs. AACN monitored the Expert Panel's work to ensure that the competencies would apply to both NP and CNS practices. The Validation Panel's task was to evaluate the work of the Expert Panel by performing a systematic review of each competency with regard to its comprehensiveness, relevance, and specificity. An overwhelming consensus on the competencies was reached by the Validation Panel.

Relationship to Other APN Competency Documents

The AACN/JAHF Competencies is intended to complement, not replace, other APN competency documents. Its purpose is to bring to light the evidence-based knowledge and competencies that are essential for all APNs who provide care for older adults. In fact, these competencies build on other APN competency documents, including the Domains and Competencies of Nurse Practitioner Practice (NONPF, 2002) and the Statement on Clinical Nurse Specialist Practice and Education (NACNS, 2004). A discussion of these APN competency documents follows.

The Domains and Competencies of Nurse Practitioner Practice (NONPF, 2002) is the product of a collaborative effort by NONPF and AACN with funding provided by the Division of Nursing. Initially created by NONPF in 1990 and revised in 1995 and 2000, the domains provide a theoretical framework for NP practice. A growing national demand for competency-driven education provided the impetus for the creation of NONPF in 2002. In addition to the NONPF NP core competencies, this document includes entry-level competencies, within the context of the NONPF Domains for NP practice, for five NP specialty areas: adult, family, gerontological, pediatric, and women's health primary care. A consensus-building process was used in the development of these competencies. The aim of this competency document was its intended use as a national standard in the development of NP curricula and programs for the five NP specialty areas, and to serve as a model for future development of other specialty-focused NP roles (NONPF, 2002). Since the publication of the AACN/JAHF Competencies in 2004, NONPF has revised the Domains and Competencies of Nurse Practitioner Practice (NONPF, 2006). This revision was the result of feedback from NP faculty related to redundancy within the document and the large number of competencies. Even though there were significant revisions in the language and structure of the content in NONPF 2006, the content itself was not changed (NONPF, 2006).

The NACNS publication, *Statement on Clinical Nurse Specialist Practice and Education* (NACNS, 2004), provides the basis for CNS practice. It consists of three "Spheres of Influence," for which outcomes and core competencies are defined. The core competencies are generic, not specialty-focused, and apply to the practice of all CNSs. They describe the distinctive contributions of CNSs to health care and help differentiate CNS practice from the practice of other APNs (AACN, 2004). The Organizing Framework

TABLE 6.1. Selected AACN/JAHF Competencies

Competency No.	Description
1.	Differentiate normal aging from illness and disease processes.
6.	Assess older adult's, family's, and caregiver's abilities to execute plans of care.
11.	Identify signs and symptoms indicative of change in mental status, e.g., agitation, anxiety, depression, substance use, delirium, and dementia.
17.	Maintain or maximize muscle function and mobility, continence, mood, memory and orientation, nutrition, and hydration.
23.	Review treatment options and facilitate decision making with the patient, family, and other caregivers or the patient's health care proxy.
33.	Promote continuity of care and manage transitions across the continuum of care.
37.	Address the impact of agism, sexism, and cultural biases on health care policies and systems.
45.	Adapt age-specific assessment methods or tools to a culturally diverse population.

Source: Adapted from American Association of Colleges (AACN). (2004). *Nurse Practitioner and Clinical Nurse Specialist Competencies for Older Adult Care.* Washington, DC: Author.

and Core Competencies for CNSs have undergone a recent revision, and may be found on the NACNS Web site at http://www.nacns.org/Educators/ResourcesforEducators/tabid/139/Default.aspx.

Description of the AACN/JAHF Competencies

The AACN/JAHF Competencies consists of 47 entry-level competencies for graduates of nongerontological APN programs that prepare students to provide care to older adults. These competencies are not intended to address the specialized and complex care delivered by gerontological NPs or CNSs. Instead, their purpose is to call attention to the differences in older adults with regard to disease presentation, treatment approaches, and responses to treatment. They are not role specific, and address the areas of care of older adults that are common to both nongerontological NPs and CNSs, nor are they specialty or practice-setting specific. Because they are so general, some of them may be found in other APN core or specialty competency documents (AACN, 2004). Selected competencies are found in Table 6.1 and the entire list is in Appendix A.

A Tool for the Integration of Gerontological Content

A primary intent of the AACN/JAHF Competencies was that it would be useful as a tool for the integration of gerontological content into nongerontological APN programs. In order to assist faculty in this task, the 47 competencies were incorporated into the NONPF 2002 NP Domains and the NACNS 2004 Spheres of Influence. In both the NP and CNS documents, the AACN/JAHF competencies have been inserted where they were most appropriate. The text and numbering of the competencies were not changed in this process (AACN, 2004). This format provides faculty with a clear idea of where specific gerontological content should be included, and enables them to "cross-walk it" into their existing curricula. Tables 6.2 and 6.3 provide examples of this for both nongerontological NP and CNS programs, respectively. The integration of all 47 competencies the NONPF 2002 Domains is in Appendix B and the NACNS 2004 Spheres of Influence in Appendix C.

FRAMEWORK FOR INTEGRATION OF GERONTOLOGICAL CONTENT

The AACN/JAHF Competencies provides an excellent framework for integration of gerontological content into nongerontological APN curricula as already described and as shown in Tables 6.2 and 6.3 and Appendices B and C. Although the APN competency documents described previously in this chapter have undergone or are undergoing revision, the foundations and intent of the documents remain the same. Therefore, the ability to utilize the framework of the AACN/JAHF Competencies is unaffected. This section of the chapter discusses the process to be used in the integration of gerontological content and the "Integration of Gerontological Content Worksheet," a tool developed by the authors to facilitate the process (see Appendix D).

The Process

The process consists of finding answers to the following questions: (1) Which competencies need to be addressed in my program? (2) How much gerontological content is already included in my curriculum? (3) In which courses is it found? (4) What content is missing? (5) Where can it fit? (6)

TABLE 6.2. Examples of Integration of AACN/JAHF Competencies Into NONPF 2002 Domains

NONPF Domain	Related AACN/JAHF Competencies
I. Health Promotion, Health Protection, Disease Prevention, and Treatment	
A. Assessment of Health Status	3. Assess for syndromes, constellations of symptoms that may be manifestations of other health problems common to older adults, e.g., incontinence, falling, delirium, dementia, and depression.
B. Diagnosis of Health Status	9. Identify both typical and atypical manifestations of chronic and acute illnesses and diseases common to older adults.
C. Plan of Care and Implementation of Treatment	17. Maintain or maximize muscle function and mobility, continence, mood, memory and orientation, nutrition, and hydration.
II. The Nurse Practitioner–Patient Relationship	20. Account for cognitive, sensory, and perceptual problems with special attention to temperature sensation, hearing, and vision when caring for older adults.
III. The Teaching–Coaching Function	26. Educate older adults, family, and caregivers about normal vs. abnormal events, physiological changes with aging, and myths of aging.
IV. Professional Role	31. Create and enhance positive, health-promoting environments that maintain a climate of dignity and privacy for older adults.
V. Managing and Negotiating Health Care Delivery Systems	33. Promote continuity of care and manage transitions across the continuum of care.
VI. Monitoring and Ensuring the Quality of Health Care Practice	37. Address the impact of agism, sexism, and cultural biases on health care policies and systems.
VII. Cultural and Spiritual Competence	45. Adapt age-specific assessment methods or tools to a culturally diverse population.

Source: Adapted from the American Association of Colleges (AACN). (2004). *Nurse Practitioner and Clinical Nurse Specialist Competencies for Older Adult Care.* Washington, DC: Author.

TABLE 6.3. Examples of Integration of AACN/JAHF Competencies Into
NACNS Spheres of Influence

NACNS Sphere of Influence	Related AACN/JAHF Competency
I. Patient/Client	
A. Assessment	2. Use standardized assessment instruments appropriate to older adults if available, or a standardized assessment process to assess social support and health status, such as: function; cognition; mobility; pain; skin integrity; quality of life; nutrition; neglect and abuse.
B. Diagnosis, Planning, and Interventions	13. Promote and recommend immunizations and appropriate health screenings.
C. Evaluation	40. Use available technology to enhance safety and monitor the health status and outcomes of older adults.
II. Nurses and Nursing Practice	
A. Assessment	10. Recognize the presence of comorbidities and iatrogenesis in the frail older adult.
B. Diagnosis, Planning, and Interventions	28. Disseminate knowledge of skills required to care for older adults to other health care workers and caregivers through peer education, staff development, and preceptor experiences.
III. Organization/System	19. Strive for restraint-free care, minimizing the use of physical and chemical restraints, and develop the most independent and protective setting possible.

Source: Adapted from the American Association of Colleges (AACN). (2004). *Nurse Practitioner and Clinical Nurse Specialist Competencies for Older Adult Care.* Washington, DC: Author.

What learning strategies can be used? (7) What evaluation methods are appropriate? and (8) What resources will I need to accomplish this?

It is imperative to begin with the first question because the AACN/JAHF Competencies has been created for use in *all* nongerontological APN programs but not all programs will require inclusion of all 47 competencies.

For example, a pediatric NP program would most likely not be expected to include those competencies and content related to the provision of direct care to older adults. However, they may need to include those that relate to the Teaching-Coaching Function, Managing and Negotiating Health Care Delivery Systems, and Cultural and Spiritual Competence domains in situations where an older adult is the primary caregiver for the patient. Likewise, the pediatric CNS program might only include those competencies and content that directly affect the older adult caregiver's ability to provide care for the child in the home such as: number 6: Assess older adult's, family's, and caregiver's ability to execute plans of care; number 24: Consider age-related changes when executing teaching–coaching with regard to sensory and perceptual limitations, cognitive limitations, and memory changes; and number 42: Assess intergenerational differences in family members' beliefs that influence care. On the other hand, because the provision of direct care to older adults is included within the scope of practice of adult, acute and family NPs, and adult health CNSs, these programs will need to include all 47 competencies and the content related to them. Faculty in APN programs whose graduates will provide direct care to older adults in other areas of expertise, such as women's health and psychiatric mental health, will need to assess which competencies apply to their programs.

The next steps are to ascertain how much gerontological content is already included in the curriculum and in which courses it is found. This is best accomplished through a content mapping exercise in which you will thoroughly examine all course syllabi in your program for gerontological content. This content may be found, for example, listed in the topical outline for the course, in a course assignment, or as an assigned reading. Because this may be a daunting task, the creation of an ad hoc committee is suggested. Ideally, it should include faculty who teach in graduate nursing core, APN core, and specialty courses as they will be more familiar with the content of those courses. A content map will be created that is merely a table of the gerontological content included in the program and the courses in which it is found. This exercise will provide a foundation for the rest of the process and have value in enabling you to reduce content redundancy where it exists.

After these two questions have been answered, you will need to compare the results of the content mapping to the gerontological competencies deemed necessary for your program. Table 6.4 provides a sample of this type of comparison.

TABLE 6.4. Sample Comparison of Content to Gerontological Competencies

Content	Gerontological Competency
Medicare	32. Understand payment and reimbursement systems and financial resources across the continuum of care.
Health promotion for older adults	4. Assess health status and identify risk factors in older adults
	13. Promote and recommend immunizations and appropriate health screenings.
Cognition and mental status	24. Consider age-related changes when executing teaching–coaching with regard to sensory and perceptual limitations, cognitive limitations, and memory changes.
Medication safety in older adults	7. Conduct a pharmacological assessment of the older adult, including polypharmacy, drug interactions, over-the-counter and herbal product use, and ability to obtain and purchase medications, and to safely and correctly self-administer medications.
Physiological changes related to aging	1. Differentiate normal aging from illness and disease processes.
	24. Consider age-related changes when executing teaching–coaching with regard to sensory and perceptual limitations, cognitive limitations, and memory changes.
Adult learning principles	25. Utilize adult learning principles in patient, family, and caregiver education, such as timing of teaching, longer time to learn and respond, and need for individualized instruction, integration of information, and use of multiple strategies of communication.
Comorbidities	10. Recognize the presence of comorbidities and iatrogenesis in the frail older adult.
End-of-life issues	18. Use an ethical framework to address individual and family concerns about caregiving, management of pain, and end-of-life issues.
	23. Review treatment options and facilitate decision making with the patient, family, and other caregivers or the patient's health care proxy.
Evidence-based practice	36. Participate in the design and implementation of evidence-based protocols and processes of care to reduce adverse events common to older adults, such as infections, falls, and polypharmacy.

Source: Adapted from the American Association of Colleges (AACN). (2004). *Nurse Practitioner and Clinical Nurse Specialist Competencies for Older Adult Care.* Washington, DC: Author.

This comparison will allow you to assess which competencies are already being addressed in your curriculum and, indirectly, which ones are not. It will also help to lay the groundwork for the discovery of content areas that are missing and, in conjunction with the content mapping done earlier, where they may be included. Faculty in nongerontological APN programs frequently believe that it is only necessary or possible to include this content in the courses that deal specifically with clinical issues. However, as discussed in Chapter 3: Gerontological Content That Needs to Be Included, there is an abundance of essential content that fits well in some of the more traditional graduate nursing core courses such as theory and health policy. The integration of gerontological content into graduate nursing core, APN core, and specialty courses is discussed at length in Chapters 7, 8, and 9, respectively. Content to be included as well as strategies to facilitate the process are addressed.

Once you have determined what content needs to be included, you will need to focus on the learning strategies that can be used to accomplish the task and the evaluation of learner outcomes. Chapter 2 discussed challenges to the inclusion of gerontological content and provided a wealth of strategies to overcome these challenges. In addition, the learning strategies that you have used for nongerontological content work just as well for gerontological content. As with other content, the evaluation methods to assess learning outcomes for the gerontological content will depend upon the learning strategies that you have used. Multiple-choice exams, case study methodology, papers, oral presentations, and participation in discussion boards on the academic learning management system subscribed to by your university are all suitable methods of evaluation.

The question regarding resources may pose the greatest challenge, especially if there is not a gerontological presence at your school or university. In addition to the detailed annotated lists of print media and Internet resources presented in Chapters 4 and 5, there are other resources highlighted in Chapters 7, 8, and 9. You can also extend your reach by seeking out gerontological expertise, such as geriatricians, gerontological APNs, and geriatric social workers, either locally or regionally, to serve as consultants or guest lecturers. Other virtually untapped resources are the older adults who live and work in your community and who will be the patients for whom your graduates will provide care. The content and perspective that they will bring to the classroom is unparalleled.

Integration of Gerontological Content Worksheet

The worksheet was initially developed for use at a 3-hour workshop at a national NP meeting (Duffy, Auerhahn, & Kennedy-Malone, 2009). Workshop participants' feedback about the Worksheet was overwhelmingly positive. As a result, it has been modified and expanded by the authors for this text.

The worksheet consists of a table with the following columns: course, content, competencies, learning strategies, and evaluation methods (see Appendix D). To facilitate the use of the worksheet, you may recreate it in a Word document and save it on your computer. The course names used in the worksheet are only intended to serve as examples. They may be changed to more accurately reflect the courses in your program.

The worksheet can be used throughout the process, beginning by entering the information obtained from the content mapping and comparison to the competencies in the appropriate columns. Learning strategies and evaluation methods being used in these courses for this content can then be added. Table 6.5 presents a model of how selected areas from Table 6.4 are entered into the worksheet with learning strategies and evaluation methods added. As additional content, related competencies, and appropriate course locations are identified, they can be entered into the worksheet. Learning strategies and evaluation methods can then be selected and entered as well. When this is completed, you will have a competency-based blueprint for the integration of gerontological content into your APN curriculum.

SUMMARY

Competencies provide the foundation for APN education and practice. Their intent is to create consistency in program content, expected student outcomes, and practice standards. Although there are various APN competency documents, their intent is comparable to one another and they have a common goal of ensuring the delivery of safe, comprehensive patient care. They are not stagnant, and undergo review and revision as needed on a regular basis. The changing population demographics in this country have prompted a review and revision of some of these documents. In addition, the Consensus Model for APRN Regulation (APRN & NCSBN, 2008), described in detail in Chapter 1, has included recommendations that require the integration of gerontological content in all APN programs.

TABLE 6.5. Model Use of the Worksheet

Course	Content	Competencies	Learning Strategies	Evaluation Methods
Research	Evidence-based practice	36. Participate in the design and implementation of evidence-based protocols and processes of care to reduce adverse events common to older adults, such as infections, falls, and polypharmacy.	Critique of research study with older adults	Group research project focused on common health problem in older adults
Health Promotion and Prevention Focus	Health promotion for older adults	4. Assess health status and identify risk factors in older adults. 13. Promote and recommend immunizations and appropriate health screenings.	Case studies Internet reading assignment: The Guide to Clinical Preventive Services	Oral presentation of a case multiple-choice exam questions
Health Policy	Medicare	32. Understand payment and reimbursement systems and financial resources across the continuum of care.	Internet reading assignment: CMS Website Case studies	Multiple-choice exam questions

Source: Adapted from Duffy, E., Auerhahn, C., & Kennedy-Malone, L. (2009). *Managing the Care of Older Adults: Strategies to Facilitate Nurse Practitioner Student Learning.* Presented at the National Organization of Nurse Practitioner Faculties, 35th Annual Conference, April 2009.

Within this context, and in keeping with the stated purpose of this text, "to facilitate the integration of gerontological content into curricula by faculty in nongerontological APN programs," this chapter has presented a competency-based framework for use by faculty in nongerontological APN programs. It has also presented a Worksheet that will enable faculty to develop a competency-based curriculum blueprint. Utilizing this framework and the Worksheet, Chapters 7, 8, and 9 will guide faculty through the integration process in graduate nursing core, APN core, and specialty courses.

REFERENCES

American Association of Colleges (AACN). (2004). *Nurse practitioner and clinical nurse specialist competencies for older adult care.* Washington, DC: Author.

APRN Consensus Work Group and National Council of State Boards of Nursing APRN Advisory Committee (APRN & NCSBN). (2008). *Consensus model for APRN regulation: Licensure, accreditation, certification and education.* Retrieved May 23, 2009, from www.aacn.nche.edu

Duffy, E., Auerhahn, C., & Kennedy-Malone, L. (2009). *Managing the care of older adults: Strategies to facilitate nurse practitioner student learning.* Presented at the National Organization of Nurse Practitioner Faculties, 35th Annual Conference, April 2009.

Institute of Medicine (IOM). (2003). *Health professions education: A bridge to quality board on health care services.* Washington, DC: The National Academies Press.

Mazurat, R., & Schönwetter, D. J. (2008–2009). Electronic curriculum mapping: Supporting competency-based dental education. *Journal of Canadian Dental Association, 74*(10).

National Association of Clinical Nurse Specialists. (2004). *Statement on clinical nurse specialist practice and education* (2nd ed.). Harrisburg, PA: Author.

National Organization of Nurse Practitioner Faculties and the American Association of Colleges of Nursing. (2002). *Nurse practitioner primary care competencies in specialty areas.* Washington, DC: US DHHS, HRSA, Bureau of Health Professions, Division of Nursing.

National Organization of Nurse Practitioner Faculties and the American Association of Colleges of Nursing. (2006). *Domains and core competencies of nurse practitioner practice.* Washington, DC: Author.

National Task Force on Quality Nurse Practitioner Education (NTF). (2008). *Criteria for evaluation of nurse practitioner programs.* Washington, DC: National Organization of Nurse Practitioner Faculties.

CHAPTER 7

Integration of Gerontological Content Into Graduate Nursing Core Curriculum

Carolyn Auerhahn

U tilizing the competency-based framework and process for integration of gerontological content described in Chapter 6, the next three chapters will provide guidance for the integration of this content into the different areas of the APN curriculum as defined by the Essentials of Master's Education for Advanced Practice Nursing (henceforth called Master's Essentials) (American Association of Colleges of Nursing [AACN], 1996): graduate nursing core, APN core, and specialty courses. Although the Master's Essentials are undergoing revision, most current APN programs are consistent with the 1996 version. Therefore, the use of this version in these chapters will facilitate the integration by APN faculty of gerontological content into existing courses. These chapters will include the competencies from the *Nurse Practitioner and Clinical Nurse Specialist Competencies for Older Adult Care* (AACN, 2004) that are relevant to each of the areas of the APN curriculum. They will relate back to the challenges, strategies, and gerontological content that need to be included that were featured in earlier chapters. Exemplars for integration of gerontological content into these areas will be presented as well. Examples of the use of the Integration of Gerontological Content Worksheet found in Appendix D will also be provided.

This chapter will discuss the integration of gerontological content into graduate nursing core courses, within the following content areas: research; policy, organization, and financing of health care; ethics; professional role development; theoretical foundations of nursing practice; human diversity and social issues; and health promotion and disease prevention. The content in these areas applies to all APN students regardless of their practice setting or specialty. Although this chapter is divided into sections for each of these content areas, it does not mean that there needs to be a course for each of them (AACN, 1996). It is entirely possible, and highly likely, that some of the content areas are grouped into a single course, such as research and theory or ethics and human diversity and social issues.

RESEARCH

In APN education, the research component of the graduate nursing core plays a critical role in developing an evidence-based foundation for practice. APN students need to learn how to evaluate research, identify clinical problems and practice outcomes within the practice setting, and incorporate research findings into their practice with the ultimate goals of delivering high-quality care and improving practice (AACN, 1996). The competencies (AACN, 2004) that are relevant to these outcomes are: 36. Participate in the design and implementation of evidence-based protocols and processes of care to reduce adverse events common to older adults, such as infections, falls, and polypharmacy; 38. Use public and private databases to incorporate evidence-based practices into the care of older adults; and 39. Apply evidence-based practice using quality improvement methodologies in providing quality care to older adults.

The basic content that needs to be included in the research component and the teaching/learning strategies employed are the same regardless of specialty. The differences and, perhaps, the challenges lie in the application of this content to the older adult population. There are age-related differences encountered in research with older adults that must be acknowledged, discussed, and made the focus of teaching/learning activities. For example, there are as likely to be differences in design, sampling strategies, informed consent, and expected outcomes when the research subjects are older adults as there are when they are children. Strategies that can be utilized in this task and to evaluate the achievement of the relevant competencies include assigned readings, case studies, test questions, and written assignments.

The selection of research articles specific to older adults for critique either in class or as a take-home assignment (Kohlenberg, Kennedy-Malone, Crane, & Letvak, 2007), classroom discussions of recruitment issues in research with older adults, and the use of case studies related to informed consent with older adults (Kennedy-Malone et al., 2006) are examples of successful teaching/learning activities for the integration of gerontological content into the research component of the graduate nursing core. Another example is an individual or group assignment related to practice protocols that are specific to older adults. The assignment may involve a critique of an established evidence-based protocol (Kennedy-Malone et al., 2006) or of a policy or procedure currently being used in a student's practice site (Kohlenberg et al., 2007).

Sources for evidence-based protocols include *Evidence-Based Geriatric Nursing Protocols for Best Practice*, Third Edition (Capezuti, Zwicker, Mezey, & Fulmer, 2008), *Critical Care Nursing of Older Adults: Best Practices*, Third Edition (Foreman, Milisen, & Fulmer, 2009), and the *Try This:*® series (Hartford Institute for Geriatric Nursing [HIGN], 2009). In addition, peer-reviewed journals that focus on gerontology, such as *Geriatric Nursing*, the *Journal of Gerontological Nursing*, *Research in Gerontological Nursing*, and the *Journal of the American Geriatrics Society*, are good resources for evidence-based protocols and research articles.

POLICY, ORGANIZATION, AND FINANCING OF HEALTH CARE

The organization and financing of health care have become "moving targets," with health care policy struggling to keep up with the changes. In order to provide quality, cost-effective care within this rapidly changing environment, APN students need to develop a comprehensive knowledge base regarding health care policy, an understanding of the process involved, and its impact on health care delivery (AACN, 1996). They must be able to analyze the results of relevant policy research, to understand the context of legislative versus regulatory policy, the interaction between regulatory controls and quality controls in health care, and to evaluate health care policy issues and trends at the local, state, and national levels (AACN, 1996). They also need to develop a full appreciation for the ways in which health care is organized, delivered, and financed across the continuum of health care settings (AACN, 1996).

The competencies (AACN, 2004) that are relevant to health care policy outcomes for APN students are: 29. Advocate within the health care system and policy arenas for the health needs of older adults, especially the frail and markedly advanced older adult; and 37. Address the impact of agism, sexism, and cultural biases on health care policies and systems. Those specific to the organization of the health care delivery system outcomes are: 19. Strive for restraint-free care, minimizing the use of physical and chemical restraints, and develop the most independent and protective setting possible; 31. Create and enhance positive, health-promoting environments that maintain a climate of dignity and privacy for older adults; 33. Promote continuity of care and manage transitions across the continuum of care; 40. Use available technology to enhance safety and monitor the health status and outcomes of older adults; and 41. Facilitate access to hospice and palliative care to maximize a peaceful, pain-free, and compassionate death for patients with any end-stage disease, including dementia. There is one competency—number 32. Understand payment and reimbursement systems and financial resources across the continuum of care—that is relevant to heath care financing outcomes.

In addition to the basic content applicable for all APN students included in this component of the graduate nursing core, there are two broad areas of gerontological content that must be included: demography and epidemiology of aging, including the growth and heterogeneity of the older adult population and the mechanisms and implications of health care policies and financing for older adults. These are described in detail in Chapter 3. Resources for the gerontological content include the *Gerontological Nursing Review Syllabus*, Second Edition (Auerhahn, Capezuti, Flaherty, & Resnick, 2007), *Hazzard's Geriatric Medicine & Gerontology*, Sixth Edition (Halter, Ouslander, Tinetti, Studenski, High, & Asthana, 2009), the Centers for Medicare and Medicaid Services (CMS) Web site found at http://www.cms.hhs.gov/, the Administration on Aging (AOA) Web site found at http://www.aoa.gov/, and GeriatricWeb, which can be found at http://geriatricweb.sc.edu/.

Teaching/learning strategies that can be utilized to deliver the gerontological content and to evaluate the achievement of the relevant competencies include assigned readings both in the print media and on the Internet, in-class and online discussions, test questions, and written assignments. Examples of strategies that have been effective in delivering this content include the use of online search engines such as LexisNexis and Thomas to locate health policy documents related to care of older adults; the exploration of government regulation of care of older adults, including those related to APN regulation, in either classroom or written assignments; and an assignment in which students track the development of a policy related to health care for older adults (Kohlenberg et al., 2007).

ETHICS

The expansion of medical technology and other treatment innovations has created a health care system where the demand for new services and the cost of health care delivery have soared over the last few decades. As a result, the cry for "cost containment" is coming across loud and clear and with it, expressed fears of possible health care rationing, especially in the population over age 65. Within this context arises the need for an increased emphasis on ethical decision making in all areas of health care.

The Master's Essentials clearly state that all APN programs "should develop an understanding of the principles, personal values, and beliefs that provide a framework for nursing practice . . . and should provide students the opportunity to explore their values and analyze how these values shape their professional practice and influence their decisions, and to analyze systems of health care and determine how the values underpinning them influence the interventions and care delivered" (AACN, 1996, p. 9). This is especially relevant to the care of older adults and the integration of gerontological content into nongerontological APN courses and program curricula. As discussed in Chapter 2, the lack of interest in gerontological content and the agist attitudes, beliefs, and behaviors exhibited by some students and faculty have been identified as challenges to the integration of this content. It is vital that APN students develop knowledge and skills to enable them to identify conflicts of interest between personal, organizational, and patient viewpoints, and to propose resolutions when they occur (AACN, 1996). The competencies (AACN, 2004) that are relevant to ethical issues are: 18. Use an ethical framework to address individual and family concerns about care giving, management of pain, and end-of-life issues; 19. Strive for restraint-free care, minimizing the use of physical and chemical restraints, and develop the most independent and protective setting possible; and 23. Review treatment options and facilitate decision making with the patient, family, and other caregivers or the patient's health care proxy.

It is extremely difficult to discuss ethical issues with regard to older adults without the inclusion of legal issues, especially when addressing decision making and end-of-life care, so selected legal issues will also be included here. As discussed in Chapter 3, there are several legal and ethical issues related to older adults that must be included in all APN educational programs, such as reinforcement of compliance with Health Insurance Portability and Accountability Act (HIPAA) when caring for older adults, knowledge of the scope of power of attorney, and the legality of the different types of advance directives in individual states. Also discussed in Chapter 3 are the factors that can impact teaching/learning of ethical issues. Several excellent resources for content related to ethical and legal issues are described in Chapter 4. All of the comprehensive texts include a section on ethical and/or legal issues. *Evidence-Based Geriatric Nursing Protocols for Best Practice*, Third Edition (Capezuti et al., 2008) and *Critical Care Nursing of Older Adults: Best Practices*, Third Edition (Foreman et al., 2009) are specific for hospitalized older adults, and *Improving Hospital Care for Persons with Dementia* (Silverstein & Maslow, 2006) is specific for hospitalized older adults with dementia. *The Nurse Practitioner in Long-Term Care: Guidelines for Clinical Practice* (White & Truax, 2007) provides insight into these issues in long-term care settings. The gerontological/geriatric journals listed in Chapter 4 and the Internet resources discussed in Chapter 5 are also good sources for gerontological content related to ethical and legal issues.

Teaching/learning strategies that can be utilized to deliver the geron-tological content and to evaluate the achievement of the relevant compe-tencies include assigned readings both in print media and on the Internet, in-class and on line discussions, case studies, test questions, and written assignments. Examples of two successful strategies are the use of search engines such as LexisNexis and Thomas to find legal cases related to older adults and a written assignment of an analysis of a case study related to elder mistreatment (Kennedy-Malone et al., 2006). Classroom discussions focused on the application of ethical theories and models related to health care decision making can be a very effective method for engaging students in an exploration of their own attitudes, values, and beliefs (Kohlenberg et al., 2007).

PROFESSIONAL ROLE DEVELOPMENT

Professional role development content is an integral part of APN education that spans the didactic courses and clinical experiences throughout the cur-riculum (AACN, 1996). It is specific to and highly individualized based on specialty areas of practice. It should include content related to the nursing profession and the APN role, including requirements for and regulation of practice (AACN, 1996). Its major goal is to prepare the APN student to make the role transition from generalist nurse to APN (AACN, 1996).

This section will present this content area as it relates to the inte-gration of gerontological content into nongerontological APN programs. Within this context, the competencies (AACN, 2004) deemed relevant to professional role development are: 21. Recognize the heightened need for coordination of care with other health care providers and community resources, with special attention to the frail older adult and those with markedly advanced age; 22. Develop caring relationships with patients, families, and other caregivers to address sensitive issues, such as driving, independent living, potential for abuse, end-of-life issues, advanced directives, and finances; 28. Disseminate knowledge of skills required to care for older adults to other health care workers and caregivers through peer education, staff development, and preceptor experiences; 30. Articulate and promote to other health care providers and the public, the role within the health care team of either the NP or CNS, and its significance in improving outcomes of care for older adults; 34. Communicate to other members of the interdisciplinary care team special needs of the older adult to improve outcomes of care; and 35. Collaborate with the interdisciplinary geriatric and geropsychiatric care team to improve outcomes of care.

In addition to the basic content described in the Master's Essentials (AACN, 1996), the content related to older adults that must be included is outlined clearly in the relevant competencies listed above. Much of this content is discussed in detail in Chapter 3 and additional content resources are described in Chapters 4 and 5. The usual teaching/learning strategies can be utilized to deliver the content, but there is one strategy without which success will not be achieved—clinical experience in the care of older adults. It is absolutely essential that all APN students whose scope of practice after graduation includes older adults be placed in clinical settings that are specific to older adults, such as long-tem care facilities, house-call practices, geriatric clinics, and specialized geriatric hospital units, and where they will be assured of caring for a substantial number across the continuum of older adulthood. Although simulation technology and use in APN programs is growing rapidly, it should be viewed as supplemental to, not as a replacement for, real-life hands-on clinical experience with older adults.

THEORETICAL FOUNDATIONS OF NURSING PRACTICE

APN practice is comprehensive, holistic in approach, evidence-based, and theoretically driven (AACN, 1996). Its scientific foundation is derived not only from nursing theories but also from those of other sciences including natural, social, organizational, and biological (AACN, 1996). APN students need to gain experience in the critique and evaluation of theories and in the application of theory to practice, especially in the health care delivery system within which they will practice after graduation (AACN, 1996). Because the theoretical foundations of nursing practice are interwoven throughout the content areas in the graduate nursing core, no competencies that specifically addressed theoretical foundations were identified in the *Nurse Practitioner and Clinical Nurse Specialist Competencies for Older Adult Care* (AACN, 2004). As discussed in the research content area of this chapter, the basic content that needs to be included and the teaching/learning strategies used in this content area are the same for all specialties. It is the application of these theories to older adults that is the challenge here, as it was in research. One way that this can be accomplished is by selecting articles and research related to older adults that include an explanation of theories or theoretical concepts and engaging the APN students in a critique of their applicability to older adults (Kennedy-Malone et al., 2006). This strategy can be expanded upon in individual or group written assignments or in essay-type exam questions.

In addition to the theories that contribute to the foundation of APN practice, there are several theories related to aging that must be included when integrating gerontological content into nongerontological APN programs. These theories consist of the biochemical/molecular, cellular, genetic, and psychosocial theories of aging, which are described in detail in Chapter 3. It is important for these to be included because they not only contribute to the scientific basis for care of older adults, but they can directly have an impact on the delivery of patient care. For example, knowledge of the theory of physical aging will help the APN student to differentiate between normal changes of aging and pathological changes related to disease. The *Gerontological Nursing Review Syllabus*, Second Edition (Auerhahn et al., 2007) and *Hazzard's Geriatric Medicine & Gerontology*, Sixth Edition (Halter et al., 2009) are excellent resources for the theories of aging content. Any of the traditional teaching/learning strategies discussed in Chapter 2 are appropriate for the delivery of this content.

HUMAN DIVERSITY AND SOCIAL ISSUES

Not only is the older adult population growing in size, it is also becoming more racially and ethnically diverse. In addition, there is a clearly defined culture of aging with attendant myths and stereotypes that can impact health care delivery. Also, of equal importance are the social issues and lifestyle behaviors that cross cultural, ethnic, and racial lines and that can impact health. Within this context it is increasingly important that health care providers become more attuned to different cultural characteristics and their impact on health care (Auerhahn et al., 2007). APN programs must include content that will enable the students to develop a sense of global awareness and an understanding of the influence of culture on human behavior if they are going to be able to deliver culturally sensitive care. They must be exposed to diversity in both the classroom and clinical settings (AACN, 1996).

Competencies (AACN, 2004) that are relevant to the human diversity and social issues component of the graduate nursing core are: 42. Assess intergenerational differences in family members' beliefs that influence care, e.g., end-of-life care; 43. Recognize the potential for cultural and ethnic differences between patients and multiple caregivers to impact outcomes of care; 44. Assess patients' and caregivers' cultural and spiritual priorities as part of a holistic assessment; 45. Adapt age-specific assessment methods or tools to a culturally diverse population; 46. Educate professional and lay caregivers to provide culturally competent care to older adults; and 47. Incorporate culturally and spiritually appropriate resources into the planning and delivery of health care.

In addition to the content outlined in the Master's Essentials (AACN, 1996), the influence of culture and ethnicity on the aging process, perceptions of health and disease, and access to health care must be included, with an emphasis on the demographics of ethnic older adults in the United States, risk factors and disease prevalence in these populations, and principles for providing culturally competent health care (American Geriatrics Society [AGS], 2002). It is also necessary to include content related to lifestyle behaviors, psychosocial stressors, and coping strategies of older adults. These topics are covered in detail in Chapter 3. Any of the comprehensive texts described in Chapter 4 will be a useful resource for this content. In addition, the *Handbook of Geriatric Assessment*, Fourth Edition (Gallo, Bogner, Fulmer, & Paveza, 2006) is an excellent resource for assessment tools relevant to this content area.

Teaching/learning strategies that can be utilized to deliver the gerontological content and to evaluate the achievement of the relevant competencies include assigned readings both in print media and on the Internet, in-class and online discussions, case studies, test questions, and written assignments. Other strategies include having a group of students conduct a community assessment with a focus on the demographic makeup of older adults in the community, role-playing exercises, and inviting older adults from various cultural, ethnic, and racial groups to participate in a panel discussion about health care. Having students conduct a lifestyle assessment of older adults from different cultural, ethnic, and racial backgrounds and then present the information in the class is an ideal way to include this content.

HEALTH PROMOTION

Health promotion is an integral part of APN practice. It is one of the "value-added pieces" our patients expect from us. Health promotion for older adults has been viewed as an oxymoron until recently. The changing demographics of the older adult population, caused in part by the aging of the Baby Boomers, have contributed to this shift in perspective. Therefore, it is imperative that APN graduates have a strong theoretical and practice foundation in health promotion across the life span (AACN, 1996).

Competencies (AACN, 2004) that are relevant to health promotion for older adults are: 4. Assess health status and identify risk factors in older adults; 5. Assess the ability of the individual and family to manage developmental (life stage) transitions, resilience, and coping strategies; 13. Promote and recommend immunizations and appropriate health screenings; 14. Prevent or work to reduce common risk and environmental factors that contribute to decline in physical functional, impaired quality of life, social isolation, and excess disability in older adults; 15. Assist the patient to compensate for age-related functional changes according to chronological age groups; 17. Maintain or maximize muscle function and mobility, continence, mood, memory and orientation, nutrition, and hydration; and 27. Educate older adults, family, and caregivers about the need for preventive health care and end-of-life choices.

Content specific to health promotion for older adults that needs to be included should focus on social and lifestyle risk factors and interventions for the different levels of prevention that are specific to the health needs of older adults. This content is described in detail in Chapter 3. Two excellent text resources for content related to health promotion for older adults are *Health Promotion and Aging: Practical Applications for Health Professionals*, Fifth Edition (Haber, 2010), and *Nursing for Wellness of Older Adults*, Fifth Edition (Miller, 2009). A detailed description of each of these texts can be found in Chapter 4. A wealth of content in health promotion for older adults can also be found in the gerontological/geriatric journals and Internet resources discussed in Chapters 4 and 5, respectively.

Content delivery in the didactic courses and evaluation of achievement of the competencies is easily accomplished using the traditional teaching/learning strategies described in Chapter 2. However, the application of this content is best done in the clinical courses. In the clinical setting, APN students will have the opportunity to develop and evaluate management plans that include health promotion and counsel older adults and their

TABLE 7.1. Examples of Integration of Gerontological Content Into the Graduate Nursing Core Curriculum

Content Area	Content	Competencies	Teaching/Learning Strategies	Evaluation Methods
Research	Evidence-based practice	38. Use public and private databases to incorporate evidence-based practices into the care of older adults.	Search for and critique an established evidence-based protocol	Group project
Policy, Organization, and Financing of Health Care	Implications of health care policies for older adults	37. Address the impact of agism, sexism, and cultural biases on health care policies and systems.	Online search to locate health policy documents related to care of older adults	Written assignment
Ethics	HIPPA	23. Review treatment options and facilitate decision making with the patient, family, and other caregivers or the patient's health care proxy.	In-class discussion	Test questions
Professional Role Development	Role of APN as a member of an interdisciplinary team	35. Collaborate with the interdisciplinary geriatric and geropsychiatric care team to improve outcomes of care.	Clinical placement in a long-term care facility	Evaluation of clinical performance

(Continued)

TABLE 7.1. (*Continued*)

Content Area	Content	Competencies	Teaching/Learning Strategies	Evaluation Methods
Theoretical Foundations of Nursing Practice	Selected nursing theory	None identified	Critique for application of the theory to older adults	Written assignment
Human Diversity and Social Issues	The influence of age, culture, and ethnicity on perceptions of health and disease	42. Assesses intergenerational differences in family members' beliefs that influence care, e.g., end-of-life care	A panel discussion about health care with older adults from varying cultures	Follow-up in-class discussion
Health Promotion and Prevention Focus	Social and lifestyle and risk factors	4. Assess health status and identify risk factors in older adults.	Lifestyle assessment	Written assignment

families about healthy lifestyles (AACN, 1996). An example of a strategy that has proven to be effective is for APN students to conduct a lifestyle assessment on an older adult, identify risk factors, and develop a plan to reduce their impact on health. The in-depth nature of this assignment affords the opportunity for the student to become fully involved in the content and application of health promotion and disease prevention strategies for use in older adults. Another strategy that has proven useful is to have a group of APN students design and implement a health fair at a senior citizen center as part of their clinical practicum based upon the goals in the most recent version of Healthy People (Hamrick, Kennedy-Malone, & Barba, 2008).

SUMMARY

Within the context of a competency-based framework, this chapter has provided guidance for the integration of gerontological content into the graduate nursing core curriculum. References to detailed content and identified resources in other chapters of the book were made to provide for a more comprehensive discussion of the content included in this chapter. Examples of successful teaching/learning strategies were included as well.

To operationalize the content presented in this and the next two chapters, faculty are strongly urged to refer back to the section in Chapter 6 titled "Framework for Integration of Gerontological Content." Included in this summary is an example of the use of the Integration of Gerontological Content Worksheet discussed in that section. Table 7.1 provides an example of the use of the Worksheet for each of the content areas of the graduate nursing core curriculum.

REFERENCES

American Association of Colleges of Nursing (AACN). (1996). *The essentials of master's education for advanced practice nursing.* Washington, DC: Author.

American Association of Colleges of Nursing (AACN). (2004). *Nurse practitioner and clinical nurse specialist competencies for older adult care.* Washington, DC: Author.

American Geriatrics Society (AGS). (2002). *Areas of basic competency for the care of older patients for medical and osteopathic schools.* Retrieved from http://www.americangeriatrics.org/education/competency.shtml

Auerhahn, C., Capezuti, E., Flaherty, E., & Resnick, B. (Eds.). (2007). *Geriatric nursing review syllabus: A core curriculum in advanced practice geriatric nursing* (2nd ed.). New York: American Geriatrics Society.

Capezuti, E., Zwicker, D., Mezey, M., & Fulmer, T. (Eds.). (2008). *Evidence-based geriatric nursing protocols for best practice* (3rd ed.). New York: Springer Publishing Company.

Foreman, M. D., Milisen, K., & Fulmer, T. (Eds.). (2009). *Critical care nursing of older adults: Best practices* (3rd ed.). New York: Springer Publishing Company.

Haber, D. (2010). *Health promotion and aging: Practical applications for health professionals* (5th ed.). New York: Springer Publishing Company.

Halter, J. B., Ouslander, J. G., Tinetti, M. E., Studenski, S., High, K. P., & Asthana, S. (Eds.). (2009). *Hazzard's geriatric medicine & gerontology* (6th ed.). New York: The McGraw-Hill Companies.

Hamrick, I. M., Kennedy-Malone, L., & Barba, B. (2008). Providing health care to aging North Carolinians: Educational initiatives in geriatrics. *North Carolina Medical Journal 69*(5), 383–388.

Hartford Institute for Geriatric Nursing (HIGN). (2009). *Try This:®* and *How to Try This* Series. New York: Author.

Kennedy-Malone, L., Penrod, J., Kohlenberg, E. M., Letvak, S. A., Crane, P. B., Tesh, A., Kolanowski, A., Hupcey, J., & Milone-Nuzzo, P. (2006). Integrating gerontology competencies into graduate nursing programs. *Journal of Professional Nursing, 22*(2), 123–128.

Kohlenberg, E., Kennedy-Malone, L., Crane, P., & Letvak, S. (2007). Infusing gerontological nursing content into advanced practice nursing education. *Nursing Outlook, 55,* 38–43.

Miller, C. A. (2009). *Nursing for wellness in older adults* (5th ed.). Philadelphia: Wolters Kluwer Health/Lippincott Williams & Wilkins.

Silverstein, N. M., & Maslow, K. (Eds). (2006). *Improving hospital care for persons with dementia.* New York: Springer Publishing Company.

White, B., & Truax, D. (2007). *The nurse practitioner in long-term care: Guidelines for clinical practice.* Boston: Jones and Bartlett Publishers.

Integration of Gerontological Content Into Advanced Practice Nursing Core Curriculum

Carolyn Auerhahn

The APN Core Curriculum, as defined by the Essentials of Master's Education for Advanced Practice Nursing (henceforth called Master's Essentials), applies to all APN programs whose graduates will provide direct patient care. "The purpose or outcome of the advanced practice nursing core curriculum is to prepare a graduate to assume responsibility and accountability for the health promotion, assessment, diagnosis, and management of client problems including the prescription of pharmacologic agents within a specialty area of clinical practice" (American Association of Colleges of Nursing [AACN], 1996, p. 12). The APN core curriculum consists of three specific content areas: advanced health/physical assessment; advanced physiology and pathophysiology; and advanced pharmacology. It is strongly suggested that discrete courses be created for each of these three areas in order to be able to devote ample time and focus to in-depth coverage of these critical areas of content. It is also expected that this content will continue to be included in the specialty courses (AACN, 1996).

Utilizing the competency-based framework and process for integration of gerontological content described in Chapter 6, this chapter will discuss the integration of gerontological content into the APN core curriculum as defined in the Master's Essentials. In keeping with the recommendation of the AACN (1996), it will be presented within the context of three discrete courses: Advanced Health/Physical Assessment; Advanced Physiology and Pathophysiology; and Advanced Pharmacology. Competencies from the *Nurse Practitioner and Clinical Nurse Specialist Competencies for Older*

Adult Care (AACN, 2004) that are relevant to each of these courses will be presented. Reference will be made, as appropriate, to content in earlier chapters in the text related to the challenges, strategies, and gerontological content that needs to be included. Exemplars for integration of gerontological content into these areas will also be presented. An example of the use of the Integration of Gerontological Content Worksheet found in Appendix D will also be provided.

ADVANCED HEALTH/PHYSICAL ASSESSMENT

Advanced Health/Physical Assessment is a foundational course that will be reinforced on an ongoing basis as the APN student continues into the management and clinical practicum courses. It consists of content and skills that are generic to all APN students. In addition, it may be adapted within specialty courses to include those that meet the specific needs of the various APN roles and specialties. Comprehensive and focused history and physical exam skills, as well as psychological assessment skills, are included so that the APN student will develop the ability to determine the health care strategies that are necessary and will be effective for individuals, families, and/or communities. Because effective communication skills are essential in both this course and in APN practice, the opportunity to refine and strengthen the APN student's existing communication skills must also be provided (AACN, 1996).

This section of the chapter will discuss the integration of gerontological content into the Advanced Health/Physical Assessment course. The competencies (AACN, 2004) that are relevant to advanced health/physical assessment for older adults are: 2. Use standardized assessment instruments appropriate to older adults if available, or a standardized assessment process to assess social support and health status, such as function, cognition, mobility, pain, skin integrity, quality of life, nutrition, neglect, and abuse; 11. Identify signs and symptoms indicative of change in mental status, e.g., agitation, anxiety, depression, substance use, delirium, and dementia; 12. Interpret results of appropriate laboratory and diagnostic tests, differentiating values for older adults; 44. Assess patients' and caregivers' cultural and spiritual priorities as part of a holistic assessment; and 45. Adapt age-specific assessment methods or tools to a culturally diverse population.

In addition to the basic content of this course, there are several areas of content that are specific to the assessment of older adults and must be included, especially in APN programs whose graduates' scope of practice includes older adults. A major component of this gerontological content is the Comprehensive Geriatric Assessment (CGA). In addition to the routine history, physical, and psychological assessments, a CGA includes functional status, cognitive, emotional, social, and, if indicated, nutritional assessments. A detailed discussion of CGA can be found in Chapter 3. APN students also need to develop proficiency in the basic elements of assessment using standardized instruments, such as the Geriatric Depression Scale and the Katz Index, and assessment methods, such as gait and balance assessment and recognizing normal versus abnormal signs of aging, that are specifically designed for assessment of older adults (American Geriatrics Society [AGS], 2002). Another area that must be emphasized is the adjustment that may be necessary when taking a history and/or performing a physical examination of an older adult (AGS, 2004). Detailed content about history taking, physical examination, and laboratory data interpretation for older adults is also included in Chapter 3. Two excellent resources for the gerontological content related to advanced health/physical assessment are the *Handbook of Geriatric Assessment*, Fourth Edition (Gallo, Bogner, Fulmer, & Paveza, 2006) and the *Try This:®* and *How to Try This* Series (Hartford Institute for Geriatric Nursing [HIGN], 2009). Detailed descriptions of these resources are located in Chapter 4. Internet resources include MERLOT available at www.merlot.org, GeriatricWeb available at http://geriatricweb.sc.edu/about.cfm, and POGOe available at www.pogoe.org. More information about these Web sites can be found in Chapter 5.

Teaching/learning strategies that can be utilized to deliver the gerontological content and to evaluate the achievement of the relevant competencies mirror those for other specialties and include assigned print and Internet readings, in-class discussions, case studies, hands-on practice in the clinical lab, role playing, test questions, and written assignments focused on older adults. Virginia Commonwealth University Department of Geriatrics has an excellent narrated PowerPoint presentation on functional and cognitive assessment available at https://ecurriculum.som.vcu.edu/portal/public/Functional-Cognitive-Assessment/index.html that could be an assigned reading. Another strategy that has been effective in delivering this content is the use of "geriatric" simulation mannequins (Hancock et al., 2006). Also effective is the use of the *Try This:®* and *How to Try This* Series in the clinical lab. Students will gain invaluable experience in becoming comfortable with the use of these evidence-based assessment tools.

ADVANCED PHYSIOLOGY AND PATHOPHYSIOLOGY

Coursework in advanced physiology and pathophysiology is an essential component of APN programs. It provides a foundation for assessment, clinical decision making, and disease management. The APN student must learn to identify changes in normal physiology that indicate progression toward a disease state in order to intervene appropriately. The student must also have a working knowledge of this content in order to assess response to medications. APN core content should include normal physiology, using a systems approach, and basic pathophysiology. Specialty-specific content can be included as needed in the specialty courses. As with the advanced health/physical assessment content, this content is expected to be reinforced and expanded upon in the specialty courses (AACN, 1996). Due to the extensive amount of content that must be covered, it may not be possible to limit this component of the APN core to a single course. Separate courses in advanced physiology and pathophysiology may be required. An alternative may be two courses in which the physiology and pathophysiology content are taught together but the content is divided into two parts.

This section of the chapter will discuss the integration of gerontological content into the Advanced Physiology and Pathophysiology course. The competencies (AACN, 2004) that are relevant to this course for older adults are: 1. Differentiate normal aging from illness and disease processes; and 20. Account for cognitive, sensory, and perceptual problems, with special attention to temperature sensation, hearing, and vision when caring for older adults.

In addition to the basic content in this course, there is important content that applies to older adults that must be included. The normal changes of aging, age-related changes in homeostasis, and the pathology of age-associated disease processes are essential (AGS, 2002, 2004). This content is discussed in detail in Chapter 3. There are a number of gerontological/geriatric resources described in Chapters 4 and 5 that APN faculty and students will find helpful. All of the comprehensive texts will provide the content as it applies across the continuum of care. The primary care texts are also a good resource, but the content may be restricted to primary care settings. The Internet resources detailed in Chapter 5 should all prove useful as well.

Teaching/learning strategies that can be utilized to deliver the gerontological content and to evaluate the achievement of the relevant competencies related to advanced physiology and pathophysiology are required readings, in-class lectures and discussions, case studies, test questions, and written assignments focused on older adults. Examples of successful strategies include: use of case studies focused on the impact of selected comorbidities, such as diabetes mellitus or chronic obstructive pulmonary disease, on nutritional status or infection in older adults; online discussions of age-related changes in body systems and vital organs; and written assignments focused on the comparison of normal laboratory values in younger and older adults (Kennedy-Malone et al., 2006). Another successful strategy is described in Chapter 10. It details the integration of gerontological content into a two-part pathophysiology course, and can be found in the section written by Marilyn J. Hammer, PhD, DC, RN, Assistant Professor, New York University College of Nursing.

ADVANCED PHARMACOLOGY

As with the other APN core courses, an advanced pharmacology course is an essential part of APN education. It should provide the necessary content related to basic pharmacologic principles, pharmacotherapeutics, and pharmacokinetics of a wide range of pharmaceuticals. Its content should also be integrated into the other APN core courses and throughout the specialty courses in order to provide the APN graduate with the knowledge and skills necessary for full-scope APN practice. Advanced pharmacology content is a requirement in all states in which prescriptive authority is included in the APN scope of practice (AACN, 1996).

This section of the chapter will discuss the integration of gerontological content into the Advanced Pharmacology course. The competencies (AACN, 2004) that are relevant to this course for older adults are: 7. Conduct a pharmacological assessment of the older adult, including polypharmacy, drug interactions, over-the-counter and herbal product use, and ability to obtain, purchase medications, and safely and correctly self-administer medications; and 23. Review treatment options and facilitate decision making with the patient, family, and other caregivers or the patient's health care proxy.

In addition to the required basic content in this course, there is critical content related to care of the older adult that must be included. Normal aging has a major impact on how medications are handled by the body. The axiom "start low and go slow" is one that needs to be imprinted in the minds of all APN students who provide care for older adults. Aging impacts both pharmacodynamics and pharmacokinetics and as a result, therapeutic decisions (AGS, 2002, 2004). Polypharmacy is also a major issue for older adults. Because of the high prevalence of chronic disease in people over the age of 65, the average older adult takes at least four to five prescription medications a day. In addition, medications are often prescribed to prevent certain diseases or treat common conditions such as urinary incontinence.

Added to that is the fact that a high percentage of older adults consume assorted over-the-counter medications and herbal products. As a result, they are at extremely high risk for adverse effects and drug interactions. Of interest is the recent evidence that raises the question whether there is actually more underprescribing for older adults, especially related to pain medication, than there is overprescribing. (Auerhahn, Capezuti, Flaherty, & Resnick, 2007). Other areas of concern that need to be addressed are the issues related to adherence to medication regimens and safe medication administration. Finances, cognitive impairment, adverse effects, and the use of multiple pharmacies and providers can all impact adherence and safety. Many times it is a family member or formal caregiver who is responsible for medication administration. In those cases, it is imperative that this individual be counseled in addition to the patient. Pharmacological management of older adults can be extremely complicated. Many times it just does not seem possible to reduce the number of medications an older adult is taking, but collecting detailed information from the patient and family/caregiver, collaborating with pharmacists, and keeping current on drug information may lead to a reduction in necessary medications. Resources for gerontological content on advanced pharmacology can be found in all of the comprehensive and primary care texts that are described in Chapter 4 and in the Internet resources described in Chapter 5.

Teaching/learning strategies that can be utilized to deliver the gerontological content and to evaluate the achievement of the relevant competencies for advanced pharmacology include required print and Internet readings, case studies, in-class and online discussions, test questions, and written assignments focused on older adults. There are several case studies from Virginia Commonwealth University that are available at www.virginiageriatrics.org/casestudies/pharmacotherapy/index.html that could be an assigned reading. A group assignment in which the students explore the implications of prescribing five or more medications for an older adult with regard to cost, drug–drug interactions, and age-related changes is a useful way to raise student awareness of the differences in prescribing for older adults. Another effective strategy is to require the students to read

TABLE 8.1. Examples of Integration of Gerontological Content Into the APN Core Curriculum

Content Area	Content	Competencies	Teaching/Learning Strategies	Evaluation Methods
Advanced health/ physical assessment	Comprehensive geriatric assessment	2. Use standardized assessment instruments appropriate to older adults if available, or a standardized assessment process to assess social support and health status, such as function, cognition, mobility, pain, skin integrity, quality of life, nutrition, neglect, and abuse.	Virginia Commonwealth University Department of Geriatrics PowerPoint presentation on functional and cognitive assessment	Test questions
Advanced physiology and pathophysiology	Normal changes of aging	1. Differentiate normal aging from illness and disease processes.	In-class lectures and discussions	Test questions
Advanced pharmacology	Polypharmacy	7. Conduct a pharmacological assessment of the older adult, including polypharmacy, drug interactions, over-the-counter and herbal product use, and ability to obtain and purchase medications, and safely and correctly self-administer medications.	Group assignment in which the students explore the implications of prescribing five or more medications for an older adult	Written assignment

the *Try This:®* Series Beers' Criteria for Potentially Inappropriate Medication Use in the Elderly (Hartford Institute for Geriatric Nursing [HIGN], 2009) that is available at http://hartfordign.org/trythis.

SUMMARY

Within the context of a competency-based framework, this chapter has provided guidance for the integration of gerontological content into the APN core curriculum. References to detailed content and identified resources in other chapters of the book were made to provide for a more comprehensive discussion of the content included in this chapter. Examples of successful teaching/learning strategies were included as well.

To operationalize the content presented in this chapter, faculty are strongly urged to refer back to the section in Chapter 6 entitled "Framework for Integration of Gerontological Content." Included in this summary is an example of the use of the Integration of Gerontological Content Worksheet discussed in that section. Table 8.1 provides an example of the use of the Worksheet for each of the courses in the APN core curriculum.

REFERENCES

American Association of Colleges (AACN). (1996). *The essentials of master's education for advanced practice nursing.* Washington, DC: Author.

American Association of Colleges (AACN). (2004). *Nurse practitioner and clinical nurse specialist competencies for older adult care.* Washington, DC: Author.

American Geriatrics Society (AGS). (2002). *Areas of basic competency for the care of older patients for medical and osteopathic schools.* Retrieved November 24, 2009, from http://www.americangeriatrics.org/education/competency.shtml

American Geriatrics Society Education Committee (AGS). (2004). *Curriculum guidelines for geriatrics training in internal medicine residency programs.* Retrieved November 24, 2009, from http://www.americangeriatrics.org/education/resident.shtml

Auerhahn, C., Capezuti, E., Flaherty, E., & Resnick, B. (Eds.). (2007). *Geriatric nursing review syllabus: A core curriculum in advanced practice geriatric nursing* (2nd ed.). New York: American Geriatrics Society.

Hancock, D., Helfers, M. J., Cowen, K., Letvak, S., Barba, B. E., Herrick, C., Wallace, D., Rossen, E., & Bannon, M. (2006). Integration of gerontology content in nongeriatric undergraduate nursing courses. *Geriatric Nursing, 27,* 103–111.

Hartford Institute for Geriatric Nursing (HIGN). (2009). *Try This:*® and *How to Try This* series. New York: Author.
Kennedy-Malone, L., Penrod, J., Kohlenberg, E. M, Letvak, S. A., Crane, P. B., Tesh, A., Kolanowski, A., Hupcey, J., & Milone-Nuzzo, P. (2006). Integrating gerontology competencies into graduate nursing programs. *Journal of Professional Nursing, 22*(2), 123–128.

CHAPTER 9

Integration of Gerontological Content Into Specialty Curriculum

Laurie Kennedy-Malone

The required content included in clinical management courses in APN curriculum is determined by mapping the existing national specialty competencies for functional role preparation across the courses developed by the nursing faculty in individual APN programs. In addition, nursing faculty should consider the content contained within the domains delineated in the test blueprints provided by the national certifying bodies. The determination of competency of APNs is multifaceted, requiring faculty to strategically designate evaluation criteria based on learner objectives for the course.

Ultimately, the national competencies for the distinct role-preparation and population-focused programs should be leveled across the curriculum of the individual program. Usually, specialty courses either contain a clinical component as part of the course requirement, or have a clinical practicum course that complements the didactic management course. Thus, when students are enrolled in specialty courses, their acquisition of knowledge and skills necessary to comprehensively assess a patient has already been determined. Methods to evaluate knowledge and skill-based competencies can include direct clinical observation by faculty and preceptors, participation in objective, structured clinical examinations (OSCEs), successful completion of digital learning objectives such as case studies and tutorials, and in-class exercises. Additionally, traditional methods to assess knowledge-based competencies are included, such as multiple choice-type and short-answer essay questions that are case based (Van Zuilen et al., 2008).

It is well documented that graduates from nongerontological APN programs are managing the care of older adults (Scherer, Bruce, Montgomery, & Ball, 2008; Thornlow, Auerhahn, & Stanley, 2006). However, clinical management courses currently lack content addressing atypical presentation of conditions that occur in older adults, as well specific information on syndromes and certain diseases that often present predominately in older adulthood. In this chapter, strategies will be presented to integrate gerontological content in the specialty clinical management courses. The *Nurse Practitioner and Clinical Nurse Specialist Competencies for Older Adult Care* (American Association of Colleges of Nursing [AACN], 2004) that directly relate to the content in this chapter are competencies 1–27, 32, 40–45. Appendix B and Appendix C will serve as guide for integrating gerontological content into NP and CNS curricula, respectively.

Additionally, this chapter presents an overview for APN faculty to employ to integrate gerontological content into specialty courses in nongerontological APN clinical management courses. Strategies to enhance the didactic content using gerontological E-learning objects and print media resources are addressed. Finally, creative experiential clinical learning activities and recommended clinical examinations are discussed.

GERONTOLOGIZING CLINICAL MANAGEMENT COURSES

As faculty begin the process of gerontologizing clinical management courses in APN curricula, a critical review of the current systems and focus areas already addressed in acute care, family, women's health, and psychiatric nurse practitioner clinical management courses is needed. Courses that address disease-specific presentations in nongerontological CNS programs that care for the adult patient will also need to be reviewed to determine the extent of the gerontological content in the existing courses. Additionally, curricular review should address the evaluation criteria for both the didactic and clinical components of each specialty course. It is time to move away from designating one lecture on aging and/or death and dying in the final management course in a nongerontological APN programs. Requiring content and multifaceted experiential learning activities based on the *Nurse Practitioner and Clinical Nurse Specialist Competencies for Older Adult Care* (AACN, 2004) will strengthen the capability of the graduate of APN programs to adequately care for the growing aging population.

Faculty are challenged to "embed" clinical issues of aging into the didactic and clinical course descriptions and course objectives (Hooyman, 2006) in order to prepare all students to manage the complex conditions of the aging adult. Using the overall strategies identified earlier in the book, APN faculty can begin to thread gerontological content throughout the coursework in such a way that students can perceive the care required by the older adult and, at the same time, gain an appreciation of the impact that normal aging has on the clinical management of aging patients with multiple comorbidities. By integrating gerontological content in these specialty courses, APN faculty will be able to ensure the enhancement of students' clinical decision-making ability, diagnostic reasoning, clinical management, and evaluation of care delivered to older adults.

Planning Gerontological Curricular Integration

Building upon the inclusion of gerontological content in the required pathophysiology, pharmacology, and health assessment courses, APN faculty needs to determine a seamless process to embed gerontological concepts across existing specialty courses that address the care of the adult patient. APN faculty will need to strategically review existing clinical management course materials, identifying disease conditions that are currently included under each system and focus area. Information that often goes missing in adult and life span clinical management courses pertains to the atypical presentation of diseases of older adults—conditions that predominately have initial onset in older adulthood and geriatric syndromes.

The initial step in determining how to integrate gerontological content in clinical management courses is to create a content map of the existing courses. Are the learning activities sequentially developed, building upon the gerontological knowledge and skills acquired in the APN core courses? Can the content that needs to be woven into the existing management courses be delivered via E-learning strategies in a blended curriculum program using a learning management system? What new experiential learning activities have been identified as opportunities to enhance the gerontological content? Have the curricular integration strategies identified earlier in this book been implemented to include identification of community resources and preceptors with expertise in managing the care of older adults? Finally, faculty will need to review and revise the map of existing clinical management courses to reflect the integration of gerontological content for APNs.

Shaping the Gerontological Clinical Experience

It is also critical that students receive sufficient clinical experiences with older adult patients, thus the placement of students in their practice settings needs to include continuous exposure to older adults across a variety of clinical settings in courses that address management of adult patients. Ideally, the preceptor will be someone experienced in advanced gerontological nursing or geriatric medicine. APN programs should require students to maintain a clinical log of patient encounters throughout the duration of the program. A systematic review of students' clinical logs can reveal the age range of patients that the students are examining with their preceptors. Once the faculty is familiar with the appropriateness of clinical sites that serve a predominately older adult population, it may be helpful to rotate students through these sites, especially if the preceptor has expertise in gerontological care. Faculty liaisons to the ambulatory clinical sites need to discuss with preceptors the students' need to dedicate a percentage of their clinical hours to the assessment, management, and evaluation of older adult patients in office-based practices. Encouraging APN students to use geriatric standardized assessment tools on the older adult patients and to document the findings with their preceptors will help to ensure that students are assessing older adults using developmentally appropriate instruments. Students should use required clinical guidelines in geriatric medicine and/or geriatric nursing as clinical references on site.

APN students enrolled in family, women's health, and psychiatric NP programs are often placed in a variety of community-based clinical sites to meet specific clinical objectives of the sequential management courses. Hospital-based CNSs may remain in tertiary care settings for their clinical practice, as adults older than 65 represent 30–40% of all hospitalized patients. (Newell, Raji, Lieberman, & Beach, 2004). The challenge now for APN faculty is to ensure that the students are considering the impact of normal aging on their patients when it comes to collecting accurate histories, conducting physical exams, ordering and interpreting diagnostic tests, prescribing medications, and evaluating the results of the intervention. Structuring clinical assignments for students to be cognizant of geriatric syndromes and recognizing atypical presentation of illness in older adults is another way of gerontologizing the clinical experience of nongerontological APN students.

Partnering with clinical preceptors is critical to the success of the gerontological integration. Preceptor-led activities designed to specifically address the care of the older adult should be built into the student assessment and evaluation process. As the focus shifts from taking care of an 83-year-old hospitalized patient to the care of an *older adult* with a specific condition, the student will need to focus on the impact of aging on the patient's condition.

Students are evaluated on their ability to meet specific competencies designated for the course based upon prior assessment of clinical competency in lower-level courses. With the integration of gerontological content, APN faculty who incorporate the core and specialty competencies into evaluation criteria will need to add the *Nurse Practitioner and Clinical Nurse Specialist Competencies for Older Adult Care* (AACN, 2004) to the clinical evaluation tools. These tools should be leveled based upon the student's achievement of lower-level course requirements. Preceptors will need to be familiarized with the updated tools for evaluation. The delivery of competent health care to older adults often requires consultation and referral to other health care providers and allied health professionals. Exposure to collaborative, interdisciplinary, and transdisciplinary health care teams that have expertise in managing and supporting the care of older adults is another way to enhance the gerontological preparation of family, women's health, psychiatric, and advanced practice CNSs (Futrell & Mellio, 2005). APN students could spend clinical time participating in team meetings, hospital rounds, and discharge planning sessions where the long-term care of older adults is being discussed.

Faculty should consider requiring a continuity of care clinical experience for APN students over the duration of the students' clinical coursework. Students can identify a community-dwelling older adult to visit. Initially, students can conduct a comprehensive geriatric assessment, using standardized assessment tools to gather data and establish a mutually acceptable plan of care. Tying into some of the psychosocial theories of aging, students could assist the patient in conducting a life review. Subsequent visits can include periodic medication reviews, patient education, and counseling on topics of concern to the patient. Finally, a plan for termination, along with the impact that visiting an older adult over time has had on the student, can be required for the final write-up. APN students gain the benefit of knowing one older adult patient over time, as well as familiarizing themselves with the impact of the home environment on the ability to remain independent as long as possible. Emphasis in the ongoing visits should focus on review of any health-related encounters with providers in between visits by the APN student, review of established goals, education, and counseling as needed. Faculty can request that students include an overall reflection on the continuity of care experience.

Incorporating Geriatric E-Learning Material Into Specialty Management Courses

Planning the integration of advanced gerontological content in the APN curriculum can be less burdensome if faculty already subscribe to a blended curriculum that is supported by a learning management system such as

Blackboard or Web CT. If the APN program is a distance-based program that relies heavily on a learning management system, faculty can choose to supplement existing coursework with a combination of gerontological E-learning materials designed to test the critical thinking of future health care providers (APNs as well as physicians and physician assistants) who will manage the care of older adult.

Once faculty have completed the content mapping process to note where there are deficits in the existing curriculum on content that is specific to the older adult, they can strategically determine the placement of complementary E-learning material. The challenge to faculty will be to ensure that an accurate assessment of the student's knowledge and skills of the enhanced gerontological content takes place. For instance, if students are referred to a Web site that details clinical practice guidelines specific for older adults, such as the American Geriatrics Society's *Pharmacological Management of Persistent Pain in Older Persons*, students should be tested on the material and assessed as to their competency to manage pain in older adults in the clinical setting.

Ultimately, gerontological E-learning materials selected for integration into the clinical management courses of APN curricula should be able to replace the need to add additional lectures or other synchronous methods of instruction, especially when there is a scarcity of experts available to deliver the specialized content (Ruiz, Mintzer, & Leipzig, 2006). Learning objects (case studies, tutorials, and modules) are designed to provide chunks of content that, when carefully examined by faculty, can be tied not only to the learning objectives of the course (Gainor, Goins, & Miller, 2004; Ruiz, Mintzer, & Issenberg, 2006) but directly to the specialty competencies (Thornlow et al., 2006). Faculty are challenged, however, to evaluate the overall impact of the use of blended curriculum that incorporates gerontological E-learning objects as a means of enhancing APN students' attainment of knowledge and skills needed to care for our aging population.

Selecting Geriatric Computer-Based Case Studies

Facilitating critical thinking and diagnostic reasoning using computer-based case studies is a strategy that APN faculty have long adopted. Many commercial case studies originally marketed for single or multicomputer license for an internal network are now available with direct Web access allowing for asynchronous participation outside of university computer labs. Typically, commercial case studies are purchased by schools of nursing (often with grant funding) or as a part of student course fees. There are, however, a number of Web-based gerontological clinical management cases available free for students to access via links provided by faculty in the course (learning) management system used in the delivery of hybrid courses or distance education courses.

Computer-based cases vary in complexity, challenging students to complete various components of cases, often in a step-wise format, with continuous feedback given to students on their decision making. An initial challenge to faculty is to determine the appropriateness of the cases for the courses in which the students are enrolled. Ideally, tying the components of the cases to the competencies that the students are to achieve for the course is recommended as a means of enhancing competency-based education. At the same time, requiring clinical management cases as a means of enhancing age-specific knowledge will partially fulfill the requirement of adding more gerontological content to the APN curriculum (Thornlow et al., 2006).

Five computer-based cases that students can be assigned as part of clinical management courses have been designed for APN students not specializing in gerontological nursing. These cases have been designed to afford the student the opportunity to assess an older adult patient based on the subjective and objective data provided. Students are then responsible for developing a management plan of care with the supporting rationale for the recommendations made by the APN student. The five cases studies pertain to patients with: unexplained weight loss, herpes zoster, anemia of chronic disease, pain management, and COPD (Auerhahn, 2007). Students are required to address the ongoing evaluation of the patients. The cases are tutorial in nature so that they teach content and are not designed to grade the student's work; rather, they ease faculty teaching burden of the material in the cases. The five clinical cases with content are cross-referenced to *Nurse Practitioner and Clinical Nurse Specialist Competencies for Older Adult Care* (AACN, 2004). These cases can be retrieved at the following site: http://hartfordign.org/continuing_ed/case_studies/.

A series of symptom-based case studies available for purchase in CD-ROM format for individual student use and intranet server version was designed by DxR Development Group, Inc., 20 years ago. Now in multimedia format, an option exists for students to access DxR Clinician Cases on the Web as DxR Development Group, Inc., now offers hosting of their Web-based software products. Currently, there are over 78 computer-based cases to choose from, with 18 cases pertaining to patients 65 years and older. Examples of clinical problems presented by the older adult patients include, but are not limited to: abdominal pain, blurred vision, fatigue, chest pain, weakness, headache, and dyspnea. APN faculty have the option of controlling performance standards that reflect course evaluation criteria. Students in clinical management courses should have already demonstrated competency in advanced health assessment; thus, they can be expected to complete a case in its entirety. Students are provided feedback during the patient encounter about their level of diagnostic reasoning. Another feature of the DxR cases is the ability for real-time case authoring. Faculty wishing to author their own cases can select from learning materials available from DxR Development Group, Inc.; technical support is available for authors to complete the publishing process of the case to the Web. Information on products available from DxR and brief demonstrations of cases can be accessed at http://www.dxrclinician.com/.

Geriatric Virtual Patients

An emerging technology that is being integrated into advanced nursing education is the use of virtual patients to simulate an interactive clinical setting (Skiba, 2007). A virtual patient case has been defined as "an interactive computer simulation of real-life clinical scenarios for the purpose of health professionals training, education or assessment" (Ellaway & Masters, 2008, p. 463). The use of virtual patients in medical education has been identified as a means to initially stimulate critical thinking and decision making, and at the same time facilitate the retention of information in students' long-term memory (Posel, Fleiszer, & Shore, 2009; Voelker, 2003). Integrating geriatric virtual patients into the curriculum of APNs is an excellent way to introduce students to complex problem solving that is associated with the management of geriatric patients.

Faculty considering the use of virtual patients have the option of selecting existing geriatric E-learning cases or developing cases using technology applications designed to author virtual cases. Posel, Fleiszer, and Shore provide faculty with an overview of guidelines for authoring virtual patient cases (2009). Strategies described include "matching case complexity and match it to the case objectives, include assessment and feedback from the start, support an individualized approach to learning and . . . encourage collaboration and collaborative learning" (Posel et al., 2009, pp. 703–704). While offered as the final recommendation, the selection of the authoring application to develop the case is critical to the overall success of developing and integrating the case as a learning object designed to evaluate students' abilities to critically manage and evaluate the care of a virtual geriatric patient (Posel et al., 2009).

There is a growing interest in nursing education to develop virtual worlds to simulate clinical environments using Web 2.0 technology; one such program that facilitates experiential learning is Second Life (SL). In-depth information on SL can be found on the home page (www.secondlife.com/). According to this site, SL is described as a 3-D virtual world built and owned by the end users, known as avatars (Skiba, 2007). In an article by Skiba (2009), she describes the work of nursing programs that have pioneered the use of SL to create virtual clinical centers. The up-front time to create the learning environments is time-intensive; students initially reported some hesitancy in learning how to manipulate all of the features in SL. However, the overall response from students in the programs was positive (Skiba, 2009).

An excellent resource that is available online at no cost for nursing faculty who are ready to integrate common geriatric syndromes into the advanced practice nursing curriculum are the GeriaSims products available at http://ww.pogoe.org. Nine modules developed by the University of Iowa Carver College of Medicine depict virtual patients in real-life clinical scenarios. The geriatric syndromes featured are: falls, delirium, dementia, urinary incontinence, failure to thrive, polypharmacy, functional assessment, palliative care, and ischemic stroke (Ruiz & Leipzig, 2008). According to Ruiz and Leipzig, these modules were developed with a two fold purpose, not only to introduce students to common geriatric syndromes, but to assist them in associating physiological changes with aging and clinical management. Each module allows the student the opportunity to receive immediate feedback for their selection of management choices. A "virtual mentor" is also available to answer student inquiries throughout the different sections of the computer-simulated patient chart. Faculty who wish to have more technological support for the students using GeriaSims may choose to pay a one-time fee of $250.00 by contacting geriatric-education@uiowa.edu.

If faculty are interested in creating virtual cases of older adult patients who "age" 15–20 years with increasing frailty and complexity of medical conditions, an excellent medical education resource, available for purchase for a nominal fee, has been developed by the Medical College of Wisconsin Geriatrics and Gerontology Department of Medicine through a grant from the John A. Hartford Foundation (Duthie et al., 2004). Five CD-ROMs with guidebooks are available for purchase at $25.00. Each of the five

CD-ROMs contains short video clips, 1–3 minutes in duration, of older adults in interaction with a variety of health care professionals. Geriatric E-learning objects include radiographic images and results from diagnostic studies, and assessment results from standardized geriatric assessment instruments. Family pedigrees can also be downloaded for individualized case construction. Each geriatric virtual patient has two clinical diagnoses. For faculty who would like to develop case studies or embed geriatric E- learning objects of patients from underserved ethnic minority populations, two of the patients are from ethnic minority groups. One patient is an elderly African American woman who has breast cancer and arthritis, and is facing end-of-life clinical issues; another is an older Asian American woman with osteoporosis and incontinence. One case involves an aging couple who have concerns with sexual functioning and longevity (Kerwin, 2007). The Web site with information on ordering the cases is: http://www.mcw.edu/display/docid596/GeriatricsCurriculum2.htm

Duthie and colleagues (2004) describe how their continuity case–based approach with the virtual geriatric cases was successfully embedded across the medical school curriculum. Nongeriatricians, as well as faculty teaching basic science courses such as pathophysiology and physiology, were able to use some of the clinical findings found in the cases in their courses addressing clinical conditions (Duthie et al., 2004). Nursing faculty could use a similar approach, using select aspects of each case that could "age" across the APN curriculum in the existing specialty courses in nurse practitioner and CNS programs for nongerontological students.

Use of Learning Objects to Develop Gerontological Management Resources

Identifying appropriate E-learning content in the form of digital learning objects can be a daunting task. Randomly surfing the Web for content often leads to identifying inappropriate links to content that may not be representative of the material that faculty is interested in embedding into the curriculum. Earlier in this book, Chapter 5 elaborated on a number of digital libraries that contain links to peer-reviewed resources that can be easily accessed and reused by faculty and students. For faculty with the responsibility for facilitating learning of gerontological content in the specialty courses, identifying reputable E-learning content can be a tremendous time-saver (Ruiz, Mintzer, & Issenberg, 2006). Faculty that lacks the gerontological expertise can rely on gerontological learning objects identified in the digital repositories for synchronous delivery of lectures and asynchronous modules, videos, virtual patients, and case studies that students can access via the university's learning management system (Ruiz, Mintzer, & Leipzig, 2006). As recommended previously in this book, the Portal of Geriatric Online Education (POGOe) is a free a digital repository of a growing collection of geriatric educational materials in various E-learning formats as well as a link to other geriatric and health care-related resources.

Another source for gerontological nursing learning objects that is currently under construction is the Duke Geriatric Nursing Education Learning Objects Repository (Duke Gero-LOR). According to the Web site, the Duke Gero-LOR will be a repository of open-access, digitally archived teaching and learning materials. A highlight of this repository promises to be the ability for faculty to share materials and receive feedback as to how helpful the materials are in real-world applications. Information on the Duke Gero-LOR site can be accessed at http://nursing.duke.edu/modules/son_academic/index.php?id=130.

As nursing faculty undertake the process of gerontologizing the APN curriculum, the inclusion of E-learning materials will be increasingly valuable to nongerontological nursing faculty as a means to enhance knowledge and clinical performance of APN students. Using E-learning materials, APN faculty will "become more involved as facilitators of learning and assessors of competency" (Ruiz, Mintzer, & Leipzig, 2006, p. 207). Cross-referencing the E-learning gerontological educational materials with *Nurse Practitioner and Clinical Nurse Specialist Competencies for Older Adult Care* (AACN, 2004) is the next step to ensure the attainment of gerontological competency for the APN students.

CLINICAL EVALUATION OF GERONTOLOGICAL COMPETENCY

Faculty often develop clinical evaluation tools based on national competencies for APNs. The measurement of clinical competencies is often leveled across the coursework in APN programs, building upon the knowledge and skills gained in prior courses. With the integration of gerontological nursing content to APN programs, it is essential to have evaluation tools reflect the inclusion of the specific gerontological content addressed throughout this book. Students should be evaluated in managing the care of older adults across practice settings. Ideally, the preceptor for students managing the care of older adults should be trained in advanced practice gerontological nursing or medicine, and be certified as a Gerontological NP or a board-certified geriatrician. If securing preceptors with these credentials is not feasible, it is important that the preceptor is aware of the clinical requirements for the student to complete. For instance, the students should be required to complete specialized geriatric assessment instruments on patients throughout the duration of their practicum. The findings of their assessment should be reported to the preceptor with a plan based on the findings. Additionally, the students should be evaluated based on their ability to prescribed appropriate medications for older adults and to recognize the need to alter the dosage based on diagnostic findings.

Clinical Evaluations

As mentioned previously in this chapter, expectations for clinical practicum for all APN students managing the care of older adults needs to include required exposure to older adults across clinical settings. Evaluation of students' clinical competency needs to reflect their ability to distinguish normal aging from pathology, to perform comprehensive and focused examinations utilizing appropriate standardized assessment tools, to communicate with older patients using jargon familiar to older patients, to order and interpret diagnostic studies considering the impact of normal aging, and to prescribe a therapeutic regimen reflecting age-specific recommendations.

Faculty should periodically review the clinical logs of students to determine the case mix of patients that students have been seeing with their preceptors and determine if a satisfactory number of patients are older adults and if the care provided was complex (multisystem comorbidities). Finally, faculty can develop simulated examinations inviting older adults to serve as simulated patients.

Objective Structured Clinical Examinations

Systematically assessing NP students using modified Objective Structured Clinical Examinations (OSCEs) has become a means of measuring clinical competency of students throughout the NP program (Khattab & Rawlings, 2001; Ward & Barratt, 2005). Faculty are often challenged to design simulations of common health conditions that students will likely encounter upon graduation, but with which they may have had limited experience within the actual clinical setting (Ahern-Lehmann & Rauckhorst, 2003). Inclusion of clinical scenarios that focus on conditions that commonly present in older adulthood is a means of measuring clinical competency of students enrolled in nongerontological-focused APN programs. Faculty may initially choose to develop geriatric OSCEs for teaching method, especially in programs that have not incorporated OSCEs as part of the overall clinical evaluation (Fabiny, McArdle, Peris, Inui, & Sheehan, 1998; O'Sullivan, Chao, Russell, Levine, & Fabiny, 2008).

When considering the inclusion of OSCEs into the APN program, intersperse a variety of OSCE formats in your clinical management courses. The following is a list of types of OSCEs that you can select from to develop scenarios: communication, physical examination, procedural, management, and interdisciplinary. Examples of each type of OSCE considering common clinical situations are listed in Table 9.1. When developing gerontological OSCE scenarios, faculty may choose to combine the use of human actors with high-fidelity human simulators and/or anatomical clinical trainers. One suggestion for recruiting older adult actors includes contacting a local community theater company; often, such companies have a listing of actors who may be interested in serving as simulated patients. Another avenue for identifying older adults with a desire to serve as simulated patients may be retired nursing or allied health care faculty.

When developing OSCEs to measure the student's attained clinical competency in assessing, diagnosing, managing, and/or evaluating older adults, it is imperative to know what presenting complaints have been addressed in prior coursework. Students can also be tested on procedures, diagnostic equipment, and ability to write prescriptions, as well as communicating to the patient using jargon appropriate for the educational preparation of the patient. OSCEs that involve the use of trained actors should include a component to evaluate the student's communication skills that are evaluated by the simulated patient.

In designing geriatric OSCE scenarios, consider too the various clinical settings in which students will encounter geriatric patients. Karani, Leipzig, Callahan, and Thomas (2004) describe an OSCE situation involving an older patient who is admitted to the hospital and then later discharged home. In APN programs with more than one population foci, an OSCE could be developed testing the ability of a primary care-based NP to refer to an NP who works in the acute care setting. Although not as frequently used in CNS education, geriatric OSCEs that involve multiple patient scenarios would be ideal for prioritizing care for the CNS student. Simulations using high-fidelity simulators coupled with older adult actors are particularly useful for this purpose.

TABLE 9.1. Objective Structured Clinical Examinations (OSCE): Examples of Gerontological Clinical Encounters

Type of OSCE	Clinical Situation
Communication	Delivering bad news Discussing advanced directives with a healthy older couple Planning for a transition of care
Physical examination	Differentiating between cancerous and noncancerous skin lesions and/or identification of pressure ulcers using a geriatric mannequin
	Gradual onset of central vision loss using an eye examination simulator that has a slide for age-related macular degeneration; i.e., macular exudates and subretinal hemorrhage
Procedural	Effusion of the knee: Joint aspiration using knee for aspiration simulator with an older actor presenting with a history of new onset of swelling and pain in the knee to rule out crystal-induced arthritis versus septic arthritis Dehydration in an older adult in a hypothetical nursing home situation: Obtaining a blood sample from a geriatric arm clinical trainer
	Female urinary incontinence: Use a clinical female pelvic trainer (advanced) with an older female actor complaining of urinary incontinence related to atrophic vaginitis
Management	Cough and dyspnea: High-fidelity lung simulator and an older actor complaining of recent presentation of dry cough and dyspnea
	Atrial fibrillation: High-fidelity cardiac simulator and an older actor complaining of recent presentation of palpitation and light-headedness
	Syncope versus seizure disorder: Telephone conversation with family member of a patient who sustained a fall at home.
	Apathy and irritability: Older adult actor with a new onset of depression
Interdisciplinary	Stroke rehabilitation End-of-life decisions Moderate stage Alzheimer's or Parkinson's disease Hospital admission

CURRICULAR ENHANCEMENT AND EVALUATION

The process of infusing gerontological content across the specialty courses in APN programs can be arduous and time-consuming if not carefully planned by faculty who are teaching the final courses in APN programs. The national competencies can guide the direction that faculty employ when reviewing the existing specialty courses, both the didactic as well as the clinical requirements. The initial challenge will be two fold as mentioned numerous times in this book: identifying faculty with expertise in gerontological nursing and clinical resources in the school of nursing greater community with whom APN students can be placed. The second challenge will be determining if the material that needs to be embedded into the curriculum will fit within the constraints of each approximately 15-week specialty course. The decision on how to integrate this information into the specialty courses that currently contain adult content and practicum will be individualized depending on the APN program. The recommended strategy for success is to use blended curriculum utilizing the general strategies highlighted earlier in this book as well as incorporating gerontology E-learning material. It is critical, however, to build in evaluation of the E-learning material as you do all of the currently required content.

Table 9.2 depicts a strategy to infuse gerontological content using a system approach across specialty courses identifying a variety of learning modalities that have been highlighted throughout the book.

SUMMARY

Critical to the success of embedding gerontological content in the specialty courses in APN programs will be curricular mapping of existing content and necessary identified gerontological content needed for APNs to be competent to manage the care of older adults across clinical settings. Incorporating the overall strategies recommended earlier in this book along with infusing select gerontological E-learning material into the curriculum, faculty can safely ensure that the required gerontological content for nongerontological specialties is included in APN programs. It is not enough, however, to add E-learning resources into the blended curriculum; students need to demonstrate that they "get it," as evidenced in examinations, written assignments, and all other evaluation criteria developed by the faculty. Thus, ongoing assessment of competency is critical to determine if the

TABLE 9.2. System Approach to Integrating Gerontological Content Into
APN Specialty Courses*

System of the Body	Examples of Gerontological Content With Learner Modalities to Be Integrated Into APN Specialty Courses
Head, eyes, ears, nose, and throat	Faculty to develop a module on sensory impairments using E-learning material and learning objects retrieved from POGOe
Integumentary	Computer-based: geriatric pressure ulcer case. Donald W. Reynolds Department of Geriatric Medicine at the University of Oklahoma (pressure ulcer)* http://www.ouhsc.edu/geriatricmedicine/Education/pu/ulcer.htm
	Geriatrics and the Advanced Practice Curriculum: A Series of Web-Based Interactive Case Studies. New York: Hartford Institute for Geriatric Nursing: Herpes Zoster Case http://hartfordign.org/continuing_ed/case_studies/
Cardiovascular	OSCE: Older patient with lightheadedness and palpitations who develops atrial fibrillation
Respiratory	Geriatrics and the Advanced Practice Curriculum: A Series of Web-Based Interactive Case Studies. New York: Hartford Institute for Geriatric Nursing: COPD Case http://hartfordign.org/continuing_ed/case_studies/
	Computer-based geriatric clinical management case. Virginia Commonwealth University: Respiratory System http://www.virginiageriatrics.org/casestudies/Pulm/GI/musc_gen/index.htm
Gastrointestinal	Faculty to develop a module on dysphagia using E-learning material, national clinical practice guidelines, and learning objects retrieved from POGOe
	Computer-based geriatric clinical management case. Virginia Commonwealth University: Gastrointestinal System http://www.virginiageriatrics.org/casestudies/pulmo/GI/musc/gen/index.htm
Genitourinary	Geriatric Virtual Patient: Mrs. Tang: Incontinence: Medical College of Wisconsin Geriatric Cases that "Age: Across the Curriculum. (incontinence)"* http://www.mcw.edu/display/docid596/GeriatricsCurriculum2.htm

TABLE 9.2. System Approach to Integrating Gerontological Content Into APN Specialty Courses* (*Continued*)

System of the Body	Examples of Gerontological Content With Learner Modalities to Be Integrated Into APN Specialty Courses
	Computer-based geriatric clinical management case. Virginia Commonwealth University: Women's health http://www.virginiageriatrics.org/casestudies/pulmo/GI/musc/gen/index.htm
Musculoskeletal	Computer-based geriatric rheumatology interactive case. Donald W. Reynolds Department of Geriatric Medicine at the University of Oklahoma http://www.ouhsc.edu/geriatricmedicine/Education/GeriatricRheumatology/index.htm
	Computer-based geriatric clinical management case. Virginia Commonwealth University: Musculoskeletal System http://www.virginiageriatrics.org/casestudies/Pulmo/GI/musc/_gen/index.htm
Neurological	Computer-based geriatric clinical management case. Virginia Commonwealth University: Neurological System (Dementia)* http://www.virginiageriatrics.org/casestudies/neuro_gen/index.htm
	Geriatric Virtual Patient Computer Cases: Delirium, Ischemic Stroke, Falls: The University of Iowa Geriatric Education GeriaSims (Falls, Delirium, Dementia)* http://www.healthcare.uiowa.edu/igec/resources-educators-professionals/geriasims/Default.asp
Metabolic/endocrine/ hematology	Geriatrics and the Advanced Practice Curriculum: A Series of Web-Based Interactive Case Studies. New York: Hartford Institute for Geriatric Nursing: Herpes Zoster Case
	Anemia of Chronic Disease and Unexplained Weight Loss Case http://hartfordign.org/continuing_ed/case_studies/
	Geriatric Virtual Patient: Mrs. Tang: Osteoporosis: Medical College of Wisconsin: Geriatric Cases that "Age: Across the Curriculum" http://www.mcw.edu/display/docid596/GeriatricsCurriculum2.htm

(*Continued*)

TABLE 9.2. System Approach to Integrating Gerontological Content Into APN Specialty Courses* (*Continued*)

System of the Body	Examples of Gerontological Content With Learner Modalities to Be Integrated Into APN Specialty Courses
Metabolic/endocrine/ hematology (*continued*)	Computer-based geriatric clinical management case. Virginia Commonwealth University: Thyroid Disease http://www.virginiageriatrics.org/casestudies/ micro-endo/_gen/index.htm
Psychosocial	Geriatric Virtual Patient Computer Cases: Failure to Thrive: The University of Iowa Geriatric Education GeriaSims* http://www.healthcare.uiowa.edu/igec/ resources-educators-professionals/geriasims/Default.asp

*Indicates that a geriatric syndrome is presented in the materials and/or addressed in the teaching/learning strategy.

students have attained the gerontological content. APN students also need exposure to older adult patients in a variety of clinical placements. Faculty has the option of including simulated patients in teaching experiences or in formal OSCEs to evaluate clinical competency of students. Careful ongoing assessment of students' clinical logs and review of preceptor and clinical site evaluations by students and faculty will complete the formative evaluation process. Students should be encouraged to record their gerontological experiences as part of their overall portfolio (Nierenberg et al., 2007). Following the overall curricular revision, faculty should revise both the graduate surveys and employee evaluations reflecting the inclusion of gerontological content and graduate attainment of competency.

REFERENCES

Ahern-Lehmann, C., & Rauckhorst, L. (2003). Issues in integrating problem-based learning and OSCEs into NP programs. In T. Guberski (Ed.), *New paradigms in advanced nursing practice: Teaching and technological strategies in nurse practitioner education* (pp. 9–13). Washington, DC: National Organization of Nurse Practitioner Faculties.

American Association of Colleges (AACN). (2004). *Nurse practitioner and clinical nurse specialist competencies for older adult care.* Washington, DC: Author.

Auerhahn, C. (Ed.). (2007). *Geriatrics and the advanced practice curriculum: A series of Web-based interactive case studies.* New York: Hartford Institute for Geriatric Nursing.

Duthie, E., Simpson, D., Marcdante, K., Kerwin, D., Denson, K., & Cohan, M. (2004). A collaborative strategy for reciprocal integration of basic and clinical sciences. *Journal of the International Association of Medical Science Educators, 14*(1), 34–38.

Ellaway, R., & Masters, K. (2008). AMEE Guide 32-E-Learning in medical education. Part 1: Learning, teaching, and assessment. *Medical Teacher, 30*, 455–473.

Fabiny, A., McArdle, P., Perls, T., Inui, T., & Sheehan, M. (1998). The geriatric objective structured clinical exercise: A teaching tool in a geriatrics curriculum. *Gerontology & Geriatrics Education, 18*(4), 63–70. Retrieved September 2, 2009, from CINAHL Plus with Full Text database.

Futrell, M., & Mellio, K. D. (2005). Gerontological nurse practitioners: Implications for the future. *Journal of Gerontological Nursing, 31*(4), 19–24.

Gainor, S. J., Goins, R. T., & Miller, L. A. (2004). Using online modules is a multi-modality teaching system: A high-touch high-tech approach to geriatric education. *Gerontology & Geriatrics Education, 24*(4), 45–59.

Hooyman, N. (2006). *Achieving curricular and organizational change: Impact of the CSWE geriatric enrichment in social work education project.* Alexandria, VA: Council on Social Work Education.

Karani, R., Leipzig, R., Callahan, E., & Thomas, D. (2004). An unfolding case with a linked Objective Structured Clinical Examination (OSCE): A curriculum in inpatient geriatric medicine. *Journal of the American Geriatrics Society, 52*(7), 1191–1198. Retrieved September 2, 2009, from CINAHL Plus with Full Text database.

Kerwin, D. (2007). Virtual patient case #5: Mr. & Mrs. Fred & Eleanor Clifford—chief diagnosis: functional aging. Retrieved October 14, 2009, from MedEdPORTAL http://services.aamc.org/30/mededportal/servlet/s/segment/mededportal/?subid=138

Khattab, A. D., & Rawlings, B. (2001). Assessing nurse practitioner students using a modified objective structured clinical examination (OSCE). *Nurse Education Today, 21*, 541–550.

Newell, D. A., Raji, M., Lieberman, S., & Beach, R. E. (2004) Integrating geriatric content into a medical school curriculum: Description of a successful model. *Gerontology and Geriatric Education, 25*(2), 15–32.

Nierenberg, D. W., Eliassen, M. S., McAllister, S. B., Reid, B. P., Pipas, C. F., Young, W. W., et al. (2007). A web-based system for students to document their experiences within six core competency domains during all clinical clerkships. *Academic Medicine: Journal of the Association of American Medical Colleges, 82*(1), 51–73.

O'Sullivan, P., Chao, S., Russell, M., Levine, S., & Fabiny, A. (2008). Development and implementation of an objective structured clinical examination to provide formative feedback on communication and interpersonal skills in geriatric training. *Journal of the American Geriatrics Society, 56*, 1730–1735.

Posel, N., Fleiszer, D., & Shore, B. M. (2009). 12 Tips: Guidelines for authoring virtual patient cases. *Medical Teacher, 31*(8), 701–708.

Ruiz, J. G., & Leipzig, R. M. (2008). GeriaSims: Falls module. *Journal of the American Geriatrics Society, 56*(1), 130–131.

Ruiz, J. G., Mintzer, M. J., & Issenberg, S. B. (2006). Learning objects in medical education. *Medical Teacher, 28*(7), 599–605.

Ruiz, J., Mintzer, M. J., & Leipzig, R. M. (2006). The impact of E-learning on medical education. *Academic Medicine: Journal of the American Medical Colleges, 81*(3), 207–212.

Scherer, Y. K., Bruce, S. A., Montgomery, C. A., & Ball, L. S. (2008). A challenge in academia: Meeting the healthcare needs of the growing number of older adults. *Journal of the American Academy of Nurse Practitioners, 20*(9), 471–476.

Skiba, D. J. (2007). Emerging technologies center: Nursing education 2.0: A second life. *Nursing Education Perspectives, 28*(3), 156–157.

Skiba, D. J. (2009). Emerging technologies center: Nursing education 2.0: A second look at a second life. *Nursing Education Perspectives, 30*(2), 129–131.

Thornlow, D. K., Auerhahn, C., & Stanley, J. (2006). A necessity not a luxury: Preparing advanced practice nurses to care for older adults. *Journal of Professional Nursing, 22*(2), 116–122.

Ward, H., & Barratt, J. (2005). Assessment of nurse practitioner advanced clinical practice skills: Using the objective structured clinical examination (OSCE). *Primary Health Care, 15*(10), 37–41. Retrieved September 2, 2009, from CINAHL Plus with Full Text database.

Van Zuilen, M. H., Mintzer, M. J., Milanez, M. N., Kaiser, R. M., Rodriguez, O., Paniagua, M. A., et al. (2008). A competency-based medical student curriculum targeting key geriatric syndromes. *Gerontology & Geriatrics Education, 28*(3), 29–45.

Voelker, R. (2003). Virtual patients help medical students link basic science with clinical care. *Journal of the American Medical Association, 290*, 1700–1701.

CHAPTER 10

"Success Stories"

Carolyn Auerhahn

Caroline Dorsen

Marilyn J. Hammer

Kathleen Meyer

Leslie-Faith Morritt Taub

M. Catherine Wollman

The final chapter of this text comprises content solicited from APN faculty who have been successful in integrating gerontological content into courses that are not expressly gerontological APN courses. The chapter is divided into two sections. The first consists of exemplars or "success stories" that clearly demonstrate how integration of gerontological content into individual nongerontological APN courses can be accomplished. The second section contains one "success story" that presents the integration of diabetes mellitus (DM) into three sequential courses in an adult gerontological NP program. Beginning with content related to the diagnosis and management of DM within the context of the entire adult population in the first course, it then presents this content specifically as it relates to community-dwelling older adults and then to complex, frail, older adults with multiple comorbidities in the second and third courses. Utilizing DM as a prototype, it serves as a model for the integration of gerontological content related to chronic disease management. Although the "success story" presented here is for an adult gerontological NP program, it can easily be applied in nongerontological APN programs. Each of the exemplars contains content in the following areas: description of the course and its placement within the curriculum; gerontological content that was emphasized and strategies used for its integration into the course; expected student outcomes and how they were measured; any challenges encountered and strategies used to overcome them; and resources that were required and those that were used in the integration process.

EXEMPLARS OF INTEGRATION OF GERONTOLOGICAL CONTENT INTO INDIVIDUAL COURSES

New York University College of Nursing

Caroline Dorsen, MSN, FNP-BC
Clinical Instructor and Coordinator
Adult Primary Care Master's and Post Master's Programs

Course Description and Placement of the Course Within the Curriculum

Advanced Practice Nursing: Adult Primary Care is a two-semester didactic course, accompanied by a clinical practicum and seminar taken in the final year by all students in the adult, adult/palliative, adult/geriatric, and adult/holistic NP programs. Students in the geriatric NP program only take the first semester of the course. It is preceded by two didactic clinical courses focusing on health promotion, lifestyle issues, development and psychosocial issues, and differential diagnosis of common health problems across the adult life span.

Integrating APN competencies with holistic assessment, diagnostic reasoning, and analysis of differential diagnoses in primary care, the Adult Primary Care course prepares students to provide primary care to adolescents and adult clients across the life span. Students apply critical thinking and evidence-based clinical decision-making skills to develop, implement, and evaluate management plans for adolescents and adults residing in the community with acute and chronic health problems. Client advocacy, health promotion, disease prevention, and physical, functional, and mental health assessment and management are emphasized. Caseload management, interdisciplinary collaboration, community resources, and consideration of learning needs of diverse populations, clients, family, and staff are addressed.

Gerontological Content Emphasized and Integration Strategies Used

Adult Primary Care is a survey course that gives a broad overview of primary care medicine across the adult life span. To this end, until significant revisions were made to the curriculum in 2008, specific gerontological content had not historically been emphasized, but rather included in content related to the care of all adults. Although faculty clearly delineated demographics and disease trends, highlighting the disproportionate effect of disease on older adult populations, the specific presentation and management of primary care problems in elders was not formally included in the curriculum. Case studies and patient presentations in clinical seminars attempted to rectify this. However, given the growing demand for expert practitioners to care for elders in the community, faculty felt that students were not graduating with a strong enough foundation in the special care of older adults.

Thus, in 2008, faculty in the adult, adult/palliative, adult/geriatric, and adult/holistic NP programs created a task force to formulate a strategy on how to better formally include geriatric content across the curriculum. The goal of the task force was to revise the adult primary care curriculum to better prepare students in age-specific presentation and management of medical and psychosocial issues in the outpatient setting. Curriculum mapping was performed to assess the strengths and weaknesses of the program regarding care of older adults, with particular attention paid to physical assessment, pathophysiology, pharmacology, and primary care courses. Primary care content was further examined to ensure that common causes of morbidity and mortality in older populations were appropriately emphasized, and that common geriatric syndromes were included in the curriculum for all students, regardless of specialty (adult, adult/geriatric, adult/palliative or adult/holistic).

Based on the findings of the task force, the adult primary care courses were revised in three ways. First, content was added to ensure that all students had a strong foundation in gerontology. When possible, geriatric lectures were given by experts, either already on the NYU faculty or as visiting scholars from other Schools of Nursing. Secondly, readings specific to older adults in the Geriatric Nursing Review Syllabus text (Auerhahn, Capezuti, Flaherty, & Resnick, 2007) were added to already assigned readings in a general primary care textbook (Goroll & Mulley, 2008) in order to highlight the age-specific presentation and management of common primary care issues. Lastly, students were required to complete three online case studies per semester in geriatric content created by the Hartford Institute for Geriatric Nursing at New York University (NYU). These were matched to specific lectures, further emphasizing gerontological content. For example, a case study on herpes zoster was added to a general dermatology lecture, and a case study on weight loss in an elderly woman was added to a lecture on depression and anxiety in primary care.

Expected Outcomes and How They Are Measured

After completion of the Adult Primary Care course sequence, students are expected to have the skills to successfully apply the principles of primary care to diverse populations, including older adults of varying ethnic and socioeconomic backgrounds, genders, and sexual orientations. Specific outcomes related to older adults are:

1. Develop an interdisciplinary plan of primary care for adults across the life span based on theoretical knowledge and best available evidence of developmental age changes, pathophysiology and pharmacology, psychosocial development and consistent with current standards of practice.

2. Formulate differential diagnoses for actual and potential health problems for adults across the life span based on pertinent subjective and objective data.

3. Compose health teaching, health promotion, and preventive interventions for clients based on respective health beliefs and demographic variables.

4. Examine risk factors and barriers to optimal health for culturally diverse clients, their families, and their communities.

5. Choose local, regional, and national resources that support clinical decision making, consultation, advocacy, and health education needs of diverse adult populations, their families, and caregivers.

6. Analyze legal, professional, and ethical issues influencing advanced nursing practice and the primary health care delivery of adults.

Outcomes are evaluated based on two multiple-choice exams that mimic national certifying exams, informal and formal case presentations in seminar, successful completion of online geriatric content modules, and performance evaluation by clinical preceptors.

Challenges Encountered and Strategies to Overcome Them

Numerous challenges were encountered in our efforts to "gerontologize" the Adult Primary Care courses: lack of faculty expertise in geriatrics, limited financial resources, and an already overburdened schedule of topics to be covered in the adult primary care courses. Having faculty whose expertise and passions lie in the care of older adults vastly improves the content and delivery of geriatric material. However, at NYU, with the exception of the coordinator of the GNP program, none of the NP faculty are geriatric experts. Thus, we relied on existing online resources, textbooks written by experts, and the network of nursing scholars willing to give guest lectures at our university.

These resources cost little or nothing, and thus do not pose a financial burden to the College of Nursing. Lastly, by integrating readings and case studies into the existing course structure, rather than simply adding on a few lectures related to the care of older adults, we were able to ameliorate some of the concerns we had about time constraints. As well, this structure modeled to the students an integrated practice serving adults across the life span.

Resources Required

The beauty of the revisions of Adult Primary Care courses is that few additional resources are required. By using existing evidence-based, up-to-date, online information, no new faculty with geriatric expertise were needed, and thus, there were no financial repercussions for the College of Nursing, and geriatric content was integrated into the existing curriculum, rather than simply "tacked on." Students were required to purchase an additional textbook related to specific gerontological issues in primary care. However, by looking at the curriculum as a whole and making the commitment to increase geriatric content across specialties, we were able to increase collaboration among programs, and thus limit the number of additional textbook purchases required by students.

Lastly, it took a passionate commitment to gerontology by the coordinator of our GNP program to convince other faculty (whose expertise and passions lay elsewhere) that it is truly a duty, not a choice, to prepare the next generation of NPs to appropriately, skillfully, and enthusiastically treat older adults. Without her, this would not have happened at NYU.

Frances Payne Bolton School of Nursing, Case Western Reserve University

Kathleen Meyer, DNP, CNE, GCNS, BC
Instructor, Master of Science in Nursing Program

Course Description and Placement of the Course Within the Curriculum

Ethical Issues in Advanced Practice is a core course required for most of the MSN specialties. It is for one credit hour and can be taken at any place in the MSN curriculum. The focus of this course is ethical decision making for APNs and it provides a broad overview of ethical decision making at the advanced practice level. The interaction between the health care delivery system and ethical decision making for APNs is explored. Relevant ethical issues in the older adult are also explored.

Gerontological Content Emphasized and Integration Strategies Used

Content specific to older adults addresses end-of-life issues and aging in place. Consuming resources, availability of resources, long-term planning, choice, comfort, and communication are important components of the care provided by an APN to aging clients. The course begins with a basic review of principles of ethical decision making so that all students are at the same level in terms of their previous bioethics course work. Students are assigned to read *Principles of Biomedical Ethics* by Beauchamp and Childress (2001). Required readings are assigned specific to the topic for discussion. The topics that are covered either in seminar-style discussion or small-group presentations are:

1. A class on withholding and withdrawing hydration and nutrition, specifically inserting and removing gastrostomy feeding tubes and intravenous hydration, focuses on the latest evidence-based practice on comfort and quality of life. The students explore the role of the APN in counseling patients, families, and nursing staff. Relevant readings are assigned, as well as accessing the National Hospice

and Palliative Care Organization Web site (www.nhpco.org). The students examine the Clinical Practice Guidelines for Quality Palliative Care (2009) and apply the relevant guidelines to assist clients or teach staff in the best practices for ethical decision making.

2. The students review the law relating to living wills, DNRCC, (Do not resuscitate—comfort care only), DNRCC-Arrest (Do not resuscitate—comfort care only in case of arrest), and durable power of attorney for health care by reviewing Web sites that address state-specific laws and living will and power of attorney forms. They discuss the differences between full code, DNRCC, and DNRCC-Arrest and the role of the APN in counseling families and teaching staff.

3. The students discuss competency versus need for guardianship and how that determination is made. They explore the advanced practice role in assessment, staff education, and patient/family counseling about this issue. A reading assignment focuses on law related to competency and guardianship. The class discusses case studies in a seminar format.

4. The students explore the concept of aging in place, the challenges and ethical issues that evolve from a patient's desire to remain at home or in their current environment. Self-care management theory and its relationship to self-efficacy and independence are also discussed. Journal articles focused on the following topics are assigned and then discussed utilizing case studies of patients in different levels of care who are experiencing physical and cognitive changes.

   a. Resources needed to remain in the home

   b. Need for higher levels of care such as congregate meals, assisted living, and nursing home

   c. Assessment of ability to drive a motor vehicle, ADLs, and IADLs

   d. Facilitating dialogue with significant others to identify and understand needs

   e. Education of nursing staff in understanding the different levels of care and identifying by assessment a patient's need for a different level of care

   f. Understanding the resources available and needed to remain at home, both financial and in terms of caregiver needs

   g. Provide strategies to self-manage and identify resources to assist them in self-management

Outcomes Expected and How They Are Measured

The course objectives are to critically analyze the ethical issues in advanced practice nursing and integrate ethical principles into decision making. Students are expected to meet the course objectives by attending the complete intensive or every class over the semester as it is only one credit hour. Participation is required in this seminar-style course.

Course outcomes are an understanding of bioethical principles of ethical decision making and the issues that are relevant to the aging population. The student is also expected to understand the role the APN plays in ethical decision making with an aging population. The student is also expected to begin to develop an appreciation for the ethical issues facing the aging population. Outcomes are measured by class attendance, participation in seminar or small-group discussions, small-group presentation or persuasive testimony about an ethical issue, and a one-page reflection evaluating whether the course objectives were met and how the course changed their ideas about ethical decision making and the APN's role.

Challenges Encountered and the Strategies to Overcome Them

The only obstacle that has been encountered is boredom by some midwifery, anesthesia, and acute care students who have felt that the content has not been relevant to them. To address this issue, I poll the class to identify the specialties of the class and I then try to include content that is relevant to all. I do discuss the importance of the concepts to all nursing specialties.

I also review the global and national issues of aging and chronic illness, and the impact across all care settings. In some classes, I have reviewed the gerontological content in class for the seminar, but students were able to choose their own topic for a persuasive testimony assignment.

Resources Used

American College of Physicians: www.acponline.org
American Medical Association Virtual Mentor: http://virtualmentor.ama-assn.org

Beauchamp, T., & Childress, J. (2001). *Principles of biomedical ethics.* New York: Oxford University Press.
University of San Diego: www.ethics.sandiego.edu
National Hospice & Palliative Care Organization: www.nhpco.org

New York University College of Nursing

Marilyn J. Hammer, PhD, DC, RN
Assistant Professor

Course Description and Placement of the Course Within the Curriculum

Advanced Pathophysiology I and II are required courses for all clinical advanced practice nursing programs and electives for students seeking advanced degrees in nursing administration, nursing education, and nursing informatics. The courses are designed to enhance advanced practice nursing knowledge of the pathogenesis of health-related disorders throughout all stages of life. Pathophysiological processes are presented as a progressive model, incorporating normal structure and physiological function with dysfunctional states including genetic, cellular, tissue, organ, and system levels of involvement. Clinical exemplars help to solidify the scope of the pathophysiological processes.

Advanced Pathophysiology I emphasizes content related to cellular aberrations, including cancer; disorders of fluid, electrolyte, acid-base balance, and immune function; and cardiovascular, pulmonary, renal, and musculoskeletal disorders. Advanced Pathophysiology II emphasizes content related to neurology, endocrinology, gastroenterology, and reproductive disorders.

Gerontological Content Emphasized and Integration Strategies Used

Advanced Pathophysiology I and II address health issues throughout all stages of life. Discussion of disease pathogenesis in the older adult emphasizes natural physiological changes of aging including cellular senescence and, particular to the immune system, immunosenescence. Because so many disease processes involve immune system activity, understanding the role of immunosenescence is paramount.

Course content includes common disease states and how they differ within age groups. Diseases common to older adult populations that are emphasized include cancer, select types of arthritis (osteoarthritis, rheumatoid arthritis, and gouty arthritis), osteoporosis, Paget's disease, coronary heart disease, chronic obstructive pulmonary disease, renal issues, neurodegenerative changes, and issues of the endocrine system. The pathogenesis, symptoms, and long-term outcomes are discussed. Disease management strategies are briefly described, but are not the focus of these courses.

Pathophysiology I and II incorporate a number of teaching strategies. Lecture material is supported by a pathophysiology text that differentiates disease processes at varying life stages (*Pathophysiology: Concepts of Altered Health States*, Eighth Edition, by Porth and Matfin). Evidence-based information from recent studies published in peer-reviewed journals supplements textbook material and creates a rich environment for thought-provoking discussions. Additionally, weekly case studies focused on specific disease processes are posted for small group discussions. Case studies are age-specific and incorporate some of the above-mentioned diseases more frequently found in older adults. The material is further reinforced through individual article summaries on the pathophysiological process of diseases of interest within the scope of each student's advanced practice focal area. A number of students are working on their APN degrees in Geriatrics or Adult Primary Care/Geriatrics.

These advanced practice courses also aid in the development of leadership skills and collegial collaboration. Rotating leaders within each small group guide the case study discussions weekly. The group members as a whole collaborate together in answering case study questions. Students are further encouraged to bring up issues that they encounter within their work environments.

The discussions and all course materials are supported through online technology. The course Web site contains specific domains for each lecture, has open discussion boards to the class at-large, as well as private small group discussion areas. Links to various online resources for both in-class use and resources for future reference are provided.

Expected Outcomes and How They Are Measured

All expected outcomes incorporate gerontological material. These outcomes have been established by the New York University College of Nursing curriculum committee and include:

- Critically analyze changes that occur in the physiology of selected systems when they are exposed to pathogenic processes.

- Identify cellular and organ system compensatory processes in acute and chronic diseases.

- Describe physiologic and pathogenic principles to explain clinical signs and symptoms.

- Analyze the impact of environmental hazards on physiologic processes.

- Determine the physiologic basis for diagnostic testing.

- Discuss physiologic and pathogenic concepts relevant to advanced practice interventions.

- Describe the impact of pharmacologic interventions on the pathophysiology of selected disease states.

- Develop critical thinking skills related to the diagnosis and management of disease by applying principles of pathophysiology.

The class sizes of each course are large, with over 160 students per semester. Evaluation consists of two online examinations, participation in weekly case study online discussions, and one-page summaries of peer-reviewed articles about pathophysiological disease processes within the students' areas of interest. The examination content is taught through weekly lectures delivered by two co-instructors with occasional guest lecturers who are experts in specific physiological systems/disease processes. The examinations themselves include case study scenarios with associated questions on levels ranging from direct recall to application.

Challenges Encountered and Strategies to Overcome Them

The large class size is challenging in regard to creating a strong milieu for discussion, an important component for these core courses that establish a foundation of knowledge about disease processes. The online discussion boards and creating small groups of 10 students both help to overcome this challenge and allow for more intimate discussions within and among the peer groups. Additionally, most students in these courses are practicing registered nurses and bring their experiences with patients to the discussions, further enhancing the learning experience.

The structure of these courses is evolving with the incorporation of online modules that will include background material in lieu of using lecture time. These modules are currently in development, but will ultimately include information on basic cellular structure and function, refresher material on anatomy and physiology, and basic information on each disease process. This will allow the lecture to shift to more case-study discussion and application. Again, the large class size is challenging, but can be overcome through the use of audience response system technology that allows each student to electronically participate live during the lectures. This is another opportunity to further discuss the normal physiological changes of aging and how disease processes in the older adult differ from other generations.

Resources Required

Faculty with a knowledge base of pathophysiology and the influence of the normal aging process during disease states is essential. In addition to the required text, incorporation of various resources including topic experts; evidence-based information from peer-reviewed journal articles; and online resources such as the American Cancer Society, American Heart Association, American Diabetes Association, and various institutes of the National Institutes of Health supplement and enhance knowledge. Application of the material within the specialized clinical courses further solidifies the knowledge.

University of Medicine and Dentistry of New Jersey, School of Nursing

Leslie-Faith Morritt Taub, DNSc, ANP-C, GNP-BC, CDE, CBSM
Assistant Professor
Division of Graduate Studies

Course Description and Placement of the Course Within the Curriculum

Primary Care of the Adult and Aged I and II (PCAA I and II) are the first and second required clinical courses in the Adult Health, Family Health, Dual Women's Health and Adult Health, and the Dual Nurse Midwifery and Adult Health NP Programs. These courses are generally taken after Nursing Research, Advanced Pathophysiology, Clinical Skills and Physical

Diagnosis, Clinical Pharmacology, Mental Health Issues in Primary Care, and Introduction to the APN Role. For our full-time students, PCAA I and II may be taken as corequisites with some of the other courses mentioned. The focus of PCAA I and II is to develop the clinical skills and knowledge needed by primary care providers in the delivery of comprehensive health care including health promotion, health maintenance, and the diagnosis and treatment of acute and chronic illnesses in adults and the aged.

Gerontological Content Emphasized and Integration Strategies Used

PCAA I has extensive content in the areas of dermatology; ophthalmology; diseases and dysfunction of the ear, nose, and throat; respiratory illnesses; hematologic illnesses; cardiovascular diseases; and endocrine disorders. PCAA II covers content in the areas of orthopedics, rheumatology, immunology, women's health, men's health, sexually transmitted diseases, urologic problems, common psychiatric problems in primary care, and neurologic, gastrointestinal, and hepatobiliary disorders. Within each of these topics we cover how a particular disease process or age-related dysfunction (e.g., presbycusis and presbyopia) affects physical function and quality of life in the elderly. Students are introduced to evidence-based guidelines for the diagnosis and treatment of common disorders, and then there is emphasis on how they are applied or amended for gerontological patients.

Within PCAA I we require a geriatric paper to help students to synthesize the fundamental concepts of caring for elders as they apply to primary care practice. Components of the paper include age-related changes of the body systems and how these may be affected by a specific disease process or geriatric problem. Topics for this paper may include physical problems such as osteoporosis, dementia, cardiovascular disease, and arthritis. It may also include psychosocial problems such as isolation, nursing home admission, depression, bereavement/loss of a spouse, loss of independence, etc. Posted on the course Web page are all of the modules from the End of Life Curriculum for Nurse Practitioners (ELNEC), with reference lists in order to assist students who may want to choose a topic from that curriculum, such as pain management at the end of life. Within the paper the students construct a case study in which subjective and objective findings are reported. Students are encouraged to find and use assessment tools such as the Mini-Mental Status exam or the clock-drawing test for cognitive changes. Intervention and analysis are the next parts of the paper. Within these sections, students are challenged to create a management plan for the patient and then analyze how this plan would need to be changed if the patient had low literacy or was unable to pay for the medication or treatment ordered. We ask that these papers are analyses of the illness and/or sequelae as it applies to geriatric patients who may have a less-than-ideal physical, social, educational, or living situation. We challenge the student to provide optimal care in real-world situations by coming up with ideas such as: having the local pharmacist type medication instructions in large print for the sight impaired, or in Spanish for those who are not proficient in English, or provide medication with color-coded caps for those who are unable to read.

The second writing assignment in this course is a case study and three out of the five cases that can be selected are related to geriatric patients. These case studies present elders with chronic obstructive pulmonary disease (COPD), myocardial infarction (MI), and community-acquired pneumonia (CAP). The students are asked to present a brief overview of the pathophysiology, incidence, and prevalence of the disease, and a discussion of relevant factors such as the likelihood that a problem will occur in a particular age group, ethnicity, or gender. The students are also asked to discuss the impact of comorbid associations with the illness, such as an increased likelihood of an myocardial infarction in the diabetic patient. Literature searches assist the student to describe the common and uncommon symptoms of the disorder, and what particular symptoms will help in the differentiation of the diagnosis from differential diagnoses. The literature search also assists the students in outlining the expected objective findings on physical exam and what lab work or diagnostics are used to assist in making the diagnosis. We encourage students to think about a stepped approach to ordering lab work and diagnostics, and we teach them that this must be done within the parameters of only ordering tests or diagnostics that are expected to help formulate the treatment plan. For instance, screening exams such as colonoscopy would not be ordered in a patient who is not expected to have an additional 10 years of life. This training begins the process of considering the whole patient and his or her quality of life. Additionally, it encourages the process of critical thinking when applying evidence-based care to the different age groups.

In PCAA II the focus of the project is presenting a case to a preceptor, collaborating physician, or a group of colleagues. This type of presentation simulates the verbal presentation of a case. It is brief and contains only the salient information needed to make the case to support the diagnosis and plan to be proposed. The student must be prepared to add details and information that is requested by the group to support the student's diagnostic reasoning. Cases are chosen from the semester's topics and can cover such topics as Bell's palsy, herpes zoster, and bowel cancer. The student, in preparing the case, begins to understand that age, comorbidities, social history, and medications that the patient is already taking must be considered in formulating the treatment plan. In PCAA I students are introduced to the Beer's list and in this presentation they would be expected to consider medicating elders within the context of the Beer's recommendations, the problems inherent in polypharmacy, and with consideration of the aged kidney.

Expected Outcomes and How They Are Measured

Each of the papers described are uploaded onto the class Web site and they are all done as small group projects. After they are uploaded, the other students have an opportunity to ask questions, make comments, and learn from their colleagues' work. The philosophy of these courses is based on an adult learning community. Finally the papers are commented on and graded by the course leader (the didactic instructor) openly on the Web site. Clinical instructors in the course often read and comment on the papers, adding to discussion. It is in this fashion that all the students learn from each paper. The expected learning outcomes include differentiating normal age-related changes from pathological changes, how comorbid conditions of the aged may change a treatment plan, care in the use of medications to avoid polypharmacy and untoward events such as overmedication in an elder with renal insufficiency, and consideration of avoidance of medications that might contribute to falls, constipation, dehydration, dry mouth, confusion, and delirium.

Specific content is also tested throughout the semester by multiple-choice examinations. Students in PCAA I and II have clinical placements with NPs or physicians who are aware of the course objectives and provide observations and on-hand experiences that allow the student to see and then implement the geriatric concepts we teach.

Challenges Encountered and Strategies to Overcome Them

The University of Medicine and Dentistry of New Jersey School of Nursing has a second degree accelerated BSN program, 13 NP programs, and a DNP program. We provide a stand-alone course in Gerontology beginning in the BSN program, laying the foundation for future practice. Our RN students are taught that 62% of their patients will be over age 65, and that number is expected to increase as more Baby Boomers continue to age. We infuse geriatric training into our nongeriatric NP programs, and we have students who go on to develop Capstone projects with a geriatric focus such as a business proposal for establishing senior living, and a recent proposal to develop a Geriatric Emergency Department. We think that the early introduction of gerontology into our program provides a culture where our students understand that it is they who will most certainly provide care to more and more elders, and that they must become prepared at every stage of their education to take on this responsibility and develop a strong knowledge base.

Resources Required

Our School of Nursing is supported by a dedicated librarian who also is an RN. On our library Web site we have a Geriatrics Toolkit with re-sources such as geriatric databases inclusive of AgeLine (AARP, 2008), which abstracts the literature on social gerontology and age-related re-search from the fields of psychology, sociology, social work, and health sciences; DARE (National Institute for Health Research), which contains summaries of systematic reviews on a broad range of health and social top-ics; and Rehabdata (National Rehabilitation Information Center), a database that describes more than 65,000 documents covering physical, mental, and psychiatric disabilities, independent living, vocational rehabilitation, and assistive technology, to name a few. Online, we subscribe to four electronic geriatric texts such as *Reichel's Care of the Elderly* (Arenson et al., 2009) and *Geriatric Medicine: An Evidence-Based Approach* (Cassel, Leipzig, Cohen, Larson, & Meier, 2003). We subscribe to more than 23 electronic geriatric journals such as *Geriatric Nursing* and the *Journal of Aging and Health*. We provide geriatric patient information for our students to use from eight sources such as HealthyNJ (University of Medicine and Dentistry, 2009) and the National Institute on Aging—Health Information (U.S. National Institutes of Health National Institute on Aging, 2009). We have seven re-sources for PDAs including DynaMed (Ebsco, 2009), an Internet reference integrating evidence-based medicine with information for clinical practice on more than 18,000 topics, and the ePocrates suite of diagnostic, drug, and treatment tools. Included in our university resources are the New Jer-sey Institute for Successful Aging at the School of Osteopathic Medicine, and the Gerontologic Institute at Robert Wood Johnson Medical School. Finally, we provide information on selected geriatric Web resources such as the American Geriatrics Society and AgeingStats.gov, a Federal Interagency Forum on Aging-Related Statistics.

One of two NPs certified in Gerontology teaches the BSN gerontology course and a GNP also teaches half the sections of PCAA I and II. Faculty practice is encouraged to keep the faculty current and to provide clinical placements for students. Courses taught by faculty knowledgeable in geriatrics help to provide a culture where this expertise is valued.

Resources Used

AARP (2008). AgeLine, from http://star.aarp.org/cgi-bin/starfinder/0?path=ageweb
.txt&id=age1&pass=abcd&OK=OK
American Geriatrics Society. from http://www.americangeriatrics.org/
Ebsco (2009). DynaMed, from http://www.ebscohost.com/dynamed/
Epocrates. from http://www.epocrates.com/
Federal Interagency Forum on Aging Related Statistics. AgingStats.gov, from
http://www.agingstats.gov/agingstatsdotnet/main_site/default.aspx
Geriatric Nursing
Journal of Aging and Health
National Institute for Health Research. DARE (Database of Abstracts of Reviews of Effects), from http://www.crd.york.ac.uk/crdweb/Home.aspx?DB=
DARE&SessionID=&SearchID=&E=0&D=0&H=0&SearchFor=
National Rehabilitation Information Center. Rehabdata, from http://www.naric.
com/research/rehab/advanced.cfm
U.S. National Institutes of Health National Institute on Aging (2009). Health Information, from http://www.nia.nih.gov/HealthInformation/
University of Medicine and Dentistry (2009). Healthy New Jersey, from
http://www.healthynj.org/index.htm

New York University College of Nursing

Carolyn Auerhahn, EdD, ANP, GNP-BC, FAANP
Clinical Associate Professor, Coordinator Geriatric NP Programs
Associate Director and Director for Advanced Practice Initiatives, Hartford Institute for Geriatric Nursing

Course Description and Placement of the Course Within the Curriculum

Nursing Strategies: Adults and the Aged (A&A) is the first required specialty core course for the acute care, adult, adult/palliative, adult/geriatric, and geriatric NP students. It provides an introduction to theoretical, developmental, and clinical issues relevant to advanced nursing practice in the care of adults and older adults. Social, political, cultural, and ethical issues that influence access and utilization of health care are explored and health belief models are incorporated. Health promotion and disease prevention concepts and strategies are emphasized. Adult development and family theory within the context of cultural diversity are also addressed.

Gerontological Content Emphasized and Integration Strategies Used

A&A has a strong focus on aging and older adults. Content specific to older adults includes the demographics and epidemiology of aging, stereotypes and myths related to older adults, theories of aging, and the political, social, economic, and ethical issues associated with aging. Because developmental issues across the adult life span are an important part of the course, students are required to participate in a group presentation focused on one of four age groups: adolescent, young adult, middle adult, and older adult. The following areas must be covered and the content must be specific to the age group: physiological changes, psychosocial needs/tasks, and health maintenance issues/concerns. This assignment provides the students with the opportunity for an in-depth exploration of aging and the older adult.

A major emphasis of this course is health promotion and disease prevention. Health promotion content such as health screening and immunizations, risk factor concepts, lifestyle issues such as obesity and substance related disorders, determinants of health behavior, health education, and compliance in chronic illness are included. These topics are presented within the context of the entire adult life span from adolescents to older adults. Required readings for each class include those that are specific to older adults. In addition, there is a class session that addresses health promotion of the elderly. This class provides an overview of risk factors that need to be addressed by primary care providers within the context of the older adult. Nutritional issues, incontinence, constipation, physical activity, sexual activity, sleep and rest, and psychological problems including the myth of senility in old age, cognitive impairment, depression and suicide, self-concept, stress and coping are included. Also included are polypharmacy, alcohol and substance abuse, falls, and hypothermia. Social risk factors such as changes in family roles and relationships and elder mistreatment are also discussed.

One strategy that was effective is having the course taught by a GNP. If there is no GNP on the faculty, the gerontological specific content could be taught by an adjunct faculty member with gerontological expertise. Another strategy is the required texts for the course, which include *Geriatric Nursing Review Syllabus*, Second Edition, by Auerhahn et al. (*GNRS2*), and a health promotion text that covers the entire life span, *Health Promotion Throughout the Life Span*, Sixth Edition, by Edelman and Mandle, 2006. Chapters in both texts are assigned for each of the classes as appropriate. The *GNRS2* is also used in subsequent courses for the adult, adult/palliative, adult/geriatric, and geriatric NP students. Content on Web sites with a specific focus on gerontology, such as the Administration on Aging available at http://www.aoa.gov, is also assigned as required readings.

Expected Outcomes and How They Are Measured

Expected course outcomes related to the gerontological content are listed below.

- Describe current theories, concepts, and research on the aging process.

- Discuss political, social, and economic issues that affect the quality of life and quality of health care for adults throughout the life span.

- Analyze the impact of health beliefs, culture, socioeconomic status, and other determinants for health behavior on adults throughout the life span.

- Demonstrate an understanding of health promotion and disease prevention concepts and strategies relevant to adults in various stages of the life span.

- Analyze the health needs of adults in various stages of the life span.

Because the class size is approximately 80–90 students, the evaluation of these outcomes consists of two multiple-choice exams. These exams include content taught by course faculty and the group presentations.

Challenges Encountered and Strategies to Overcome Them

There was only one significant challenge encountered related to older adults: lack of student interest in gerontology content. Most of the students in the class work in the hospital setting where their experience with older adults is predominately when they are at their sickest. As a result they tend to stereotype all older adults within that context.

There were a few strategies that I used to address this challenge. I think one of the most important is that the gerontological content is presented beginning with a focus on the positive aspects of older adults, such as the high percentage of those living in the community, educational levels, and labor workforce statistics, and progressing to less-positive aspects of aging, such as theories of aging and chronic disease issues. There is also a strong wellness and healthy aging focus. Another strategy that I think has been very effective is to acknowledge the students' "bias/dislike/negative feelings" right at the beginning of the course. They seem to find it amazing that anyone would acknowledge this in an open forum. Once it is on the table it seems to lessen the impact on their learning. I also think that the attitude of the faculty toward older adults is an important factor.

Resources Required

Having faculty with gerontological expertise is essential. The gerontological content could be taught by an adjunct faculty with that expertise if there is no GNP on faculty. Inclusion of required reading assignments from gerontological texts, journal articles, and Internet sites is also essential. In addition, a proactive approach related to aging and older adults on the part of *all* faculty is the key to success.

MODEL FOR THE INTEGRATION OF GERONTOLOGICAL CONTENT IN CHRONIC DISEASE MANAGEMENT

Neumann University, Division of Nursing and Health Sciences

M. Catherine Wollman, MSN, GNP-BC
Coordinator, Adult and Geriatric NP Program

Course Description and Placement of the Course Within the Curriculum

This section will focus on the integration of Type 2 diabetes mellitus (DM) throughout three Adult Nurse Practitioner–Gerontology Nurse

Practitioner (ANP-GNP) courses. The three ANP-GNP clinical specialty courses include theory and clinical components and are taken in sequence during the last three semesters of the graduate NP curriculum. Adult-Gerontology Primary Care I focuses on primary health care of common acute and chronic health problems for adults of all ages. Adult-Gerontology Primary Care II focuses on more complex health problems including those of vulnerable older adults. In the third course, Adult-Gerontology Synthesis Practicum, the NP student integrates all aspects of the role in the management of diverse adult populations. Diabetes is integrated throughout all three clinical specialty courses with increasing complexity of content and patient management.

Gerontological Content Emphasized and Integration Strategies Used

The curriculum required to prepare NP students to provide primary care for diabetic patients is extensive and involves the full spectrum of biopsychosocial knowledge and APN skills. Additional content relevant to the unique needs of the complex and frail older diabetic is critical to provide high quality care and to improve outcomes for this more vulnerable group. By focusing on the integration of content, the student learns increasingly complex diabetic content across three courses. The NP student synthesizes initial patient management skills before they are required to manage the very complex older diabetic with multiple, severe chronic diseases.

NP educators focus a significant amount of time on content related to management of DM because of its increasing numbers in all age groups, and the complexity of acute and chronic health problems encountered by this patient population. The prevalence of DM increases with age and half of those presently diagnosed are over 60 years of age, with the highest prevalence found in those over 80 years of age (Gambert & Pinkstaff, 2006). During the first clinical specialty course, Adult-Gerontology Primary Care I, the theory and clinical focus is on the essential elements of health management for any adult with DM. The comprehensive content areas appear in Table 10.1. Clinical experiences take place in primary care offices or outpatient settings where multiple patients with DM are encountered.

In Adult-Gerontology Primary Care II, the unique challenges posed by older adults with Type 2 DM are addressed. NP students are exposed to the impact of the heterogeneity of older adult including *young old* (65–74 years), *old old* (75–84), and the *oldest old* (85 years and older). The variables in assessment and decision making for an active, community-dwelling 80-year-old and a frail 80-year-old residing in a nursing home are discussed.

TABLE 10.1. Diabetes Mellitus Curriculum for NP Students in Adult-Gerontology Primary Care I

Identification of risk factors:
- Family history/genetics
- Obesity
- Smoking
- HTN
- Hyperlipidemia
- Alcohol or substance abuse

Assessment of psychosocial issues:
- Support system
- Level of education
- Financial issues
- Sexual function

Frequency of required screenings:
- FBS
- Estimate GFR
- Microalbumin
- Monofilament screening

Age-appropriate preventive care, especially:
- Flu and pneumococcal vaccine
- Dental care

Patient self-care management plan:
- A1C goal
- SMBG schedule
- Diet
- Activity
- Tx for hypo- and hyperglycemia
- Sick days
- Medications
- Foot care
- Follow-up requirements

Review of management of cardiovascular problems (previously covered in ANP-GNP I)
- ASA or antiplatelet if appropriate
- Manage HTN
- Manage lipids
- Diet

Management of complications:
- PAD
- Peripheral neuropathy
- Pain management
- Skin breakdown

Medication management:
- Oral hypoglycemics
- Basal and bolus insulin therapies
- Patient teaching re:
  - Injection techniques
  - Equipment

Appropriate referral guidelines:
- Ophthalmology
- Podiatry
- Nephrology
- Cardiology
- Endocrinology
- Dietitian for medical nutrition therapy (MNT)
- Mental health

Content related to assessment of the older adult with DM includes a comprehensive evaluation of functional status. Areas emphasized consist of ambulation, mobility, and pain as these may all have an influence on the older adult's sense of well-being, functional status, and quality of life. Particular attention is also given to the assessment of cognition and mental status, vision, hearing, continence, gait, and balance as deficiencies in these may compromise self-care management. The Geriatric Depression Scale

(GDS), the Mini-Mental State Exam (MMSE), fall risk assessment, and other tools that are useful in the assessment of the frail older diabetic patient are introduced and the students are given the opportunity to become familiar with their use.

Other content areas relevant to the older adult with DM addressed in this course are polypharmacy and prescribing, goal setting and care planning, and community resources. Students are taught to assess for polypharmacy and its related risks using a comprehensive medication review that includes over-the-counter (OTC) medications, complementary and alternative products, alcohol, and other substances. Principles and concepts for prescribing medications and treatment regimens, including the potential differences in goals and plan of care for the active, community-dwelling 80-year-old versus the frail 80-year-old are also discussed. Content about available community resources for the older adult with a limited support system or to assist family members burdened with the stress of daily caregiving is presented as well. Exhibit 10.1 provides a summary of additional DM content related to the older adult diabetic in the second ANP-GNP Course.

In the final course, Adult-Gerontology Synthesis Practicum, student-led seminars focus on clinical situations encountered by the student. Students present case studies and are expected to include elements within the

Exhibit 10.1. Additional DM Content Reflected in Adult-Gerontology Primary Care II Course

- The frail older diabetic with altered A1C goal
- Unrecognized hypoglycemia
- Cognitive impairment
- Poor nutrition or malnutrition
- Sleep disorders
- Incontinence
- CKD, stage 3 or 4
- TIA or stroke
- Uncontrolled pain
- Sensory impairment
- Polypharmacy
- Falls or fear of falling
- Lack of support system
- Burdened caregiver
- Community resources

case study that reflect complexity of care. At this stage of clinical competence, a student will demonstrate a beginning ability to manage a complex insulin regimen in addition to management of hypertension, congestive heart failure, depression, and diabetic neuropathy. Another student may manage the diabetic with advanced dementia and prioritize the need to discuss advance directives with the patient and family or focus on palliative care and quality of life issues.

Expected Outcomes and Measurement

Students in Adult-Gerontology Primary Care I meet the following outcomes:

1. Screen and diagnose altered glucose metabolism including Type 2 DN and glucose intolerance.

2. Develop and initiate a plan of care for dietary therapy, exercise, and/or pharmacotherapeutics to manage Type 2 DM.

3. Implement evidence-based standards for clinical practice recommendations required in monitoring and managing Type 2 DM for adults.

4. Implement appropriate levels of patient education for self-management of DM.

5. Identify and refer patients for significant complications of DM.

6. Utilize a collaborative, interdisciplinary model for managing altered glucose metabolism as a chronic illness.

Students in Adult-Gerontology Primary Care II meet the following additional outcomes:

1. Collect additional assessment data related to functional status, co-morbidities, cognition, and support systems to plan care for the frail older adult with DM.

2. Utilize evidence-based strategies in the management plan of frail, chronically ill older adults with DM.

3. Include caregivers in the plan of care and teaching–learning activities when appropriate.

4. Enhance quality of life and reduce DM complications.

5. Individualize treatment to include life expectancy, level of dependence, and willingness to adhere to a treatment regimen.

Students in Adult-Gerontology Synthesis Practicum meet the following additional outcomes:

1. Demonstrate competence in critical thinking and management of the adult with DM across the continuum of care.

2. Provide quality health care for the DM patient from simple to complex.

3. Assume accountability for independent, evidence-based, and ethical advanced nursing practice as it relates to the patient with DM.

In Adult-Gerontology Primary Care I and II, students must achieve success on a multiple choice exam that includes DM content related to the course objectives. In addition, students must satisfactorily attain the clinical objectives in those courses by management of the patient with DM with minimal support. In the final Synthesis Practicum, the students' clinical case studies are evaluated and graded and students are expected to be independent with patient care management at the level of a beginning practitioner.

Challenges Encountered and Strategies to Overcome Them

The challenge that faces all NP educators is the extensive course content necessary for students to achieve beginning-level competencies as primary care providers. The integration of increasingly complex content related to management of the diabetic patient reflects a teaching strategy that allows the student to gain confidence as they manage the comprehensive care of the younger patient with Type 2 DM to the frail older adult with Type 2 DM and other multiple comorbidities.

Faculty in all courses must carefully coordinate teaching efforts in order to be successful with an integration strategy. Faculty with gerontological expertise will be more successful with the content in the second clinical course that reflects the care of the frail older adult. Faculty with even minimal gerontological expertise, however, can still be successful by using the available evidence-based guidelines for care of the older adult with DM (American Association of Clinical Endocrinologists [AACE], 2007; American Diabetes Association [ADA], 2009; Brown, Mangione, Saliba, & Sarkison, 2003; Joslin Diabetes Center and Joslin Clinic, 2007).

Resources Required

There are multiple excellent resources available to teach diabetic content to the NP student. Textbooks and journal articles are frequently updated due to the prevalence and increasing incidence of DM. Case studies and evidence-based guidelines are also available online. Excellent older adult references for DM include Brown et al. (2003) and the *Joslin Diabetes Center Guidelines for the Care of Older Adults* (2007).

In summary, the NP student will appreciate the integration of geriatric knowledge within the context of primary care management of chronic diseases including diabetes. Their ability to provide high-quality, evidence-based care will depend on their understanding of the heterogeneity of the aging population, normal aging changes, functional status, geriatric syndromes, comorbidities, frailty, caregiver issues, community resources, ethical issues, and the individual values and goals of the older person.

SUMMARY

The purpose of this text is to facilitate the integration of gerontological content into APN curricula by faculty in nongerontological APN programs. The content contained within this final chapter is consistent with that purpose. The "success stories" presented here have provided a clear direction for the integration of gerontological content into nongerontological APN programs. Exemplars for APN core and specialty courses were included. Gerontological content and strategies for its integration have been described in detail. Challenges encountered and strategies to address them have also been discussed. Necessary resources and those proven useful have been shared by the contributing authors in this chapter as well.

REFERENCES

American Association of Clinical Endocrinologists (AACE). (2007, May/June). Medical guidelines for clinical practice for the management of diabetes mellitus. *Endocrine Practice, 13*(Suppl. 1).

American Diabetes Association (ADA). (2009, January). Clinical practice recommendations. *Diabetes Care, 32*, S3-S5; doi: 10.2337/dc09-S013.

Arenson, C., Busby-Whitehead, J., Brummel-Smith, K., O'Brien, J. G., Palmer, M. H., & Reichel, W. (Eds.). (2009). *Reichel's care of the elderly* (6th ed.). New York: Cambridge University Press.

Auerhahn, C., Capezuti, E., Flaherty, E., & Resnick, B. (Eds.). (2007). *Geriatric nursing review syllabus* (2nd ed.). New York: American Geriatrics Society.

Brown, A., Mangione, C., Saliba, D., & Sarkisian, C. (2003). California Healthcare Foundation/American Geriatrics Society guidelines for improving the care of the older person with diabetes mellitus. *Journal of the American Geriatrics Society,* S1, S265–S280.

Cassel, C., Leipzig, R., Cohen, H. J., Larson, E. B., & Meier, D. E. (Eds.). (2003). *Geriatric medicine: An evidence-based approach* (4th ed.). New York: Springer-Verlag.

Edelman, C. L., & Mandle, C. L. (2006). *Health promotion throughout the life span* (6th ed.). St. Louis: Mosby

Gambert, S., & Pinkstaff, S. (2006). Emerging epidemic: Diabetes in older adults: Demography, economic impact and pathophysiology. *Diabetes Spectrum, 4*(10), 221–228.

Goroll, A. H., & Mulley, A. G. (2008). *Primary care medicine: Office evaluation and management of the adult patient* (6th ed.). Philadelphia: Lippincott Williams & Wilkins.

Joslin Diabetes Center and Joslin Clinic (Joslin). (2007). *Guideline for the care of the older adult with diabetes.* Retrieved November 22, 2009, from www.joslin.org/Files/Guideline_For_Care_Of_Older_Adults_with_Diabetes.pdf

Porth, C. M., & Matfin, G. (2008). *Pathophysiology: Concepts of altered health states* (8th ed.). Philadelphia: Wolters Kluwer Health/Lippincott Williams & Wilkins.

Nurse Practitioner and Clinical Nurse Specialist Competencies for Older Adult Care

Older adults represent a unique population, just as pediatric patients do. Consequently, the presentation of disease and response to treatment differ from other populations. The following areas of content were identified as being essential for all nurse practitioners and clinical nurse specialists caring for older adults.

For older adults, demonstrate knowledge, skills, and behavior of best practices in order to:

1. Differentiate normal aging from illness and disease processes

2. Use standardized assessment instruments appropriate to older adults if available, or a standardized assessment process to assess social support and health status, such as function, cognition, mobility, pain, skin integrity, quality of life, nutrition, neglect, and abuse

3. Assess for syndromes, constellations of symptoms that may be manifestations of other health problems common to older adults, e.g., incontinence, falling, delirium, dementia, and depression

4. Assess health status and identify risk factors in older adults

5. Assess the ability of the individual and family to manage developmental (life stage) transitions, resilience, and coping strategies

6. Assess older adult's, family's, and caregiver's ability to execute plans of care

7. Conduct a pharmacological assessment of the older adult, including polypharmacy, drug interactions, over-the-counter and herbal

product use, and ability to obtain, purchase medications, and safely and correctly self-administer medications

8. Assess for pain in the older adult, including the cognitively impaired, and develop a plan of care to manage

9. Identify both typical and atypical manifestations of chronic and acute illnesses and diseases common to older adults

10. Recognize the presence of comorbidities and iatrogenesis in the frail older adult

11. Identify signs and symptoms indicative of change in mental status, e.g., agitation, anxiety, depression, substance use, delirium, and dementia

12. Interpret results of appropriate laboratory and diagnostic tests, differentiating values for older adults

13. Promote and recommend immunizations and appropriate health screenings

14. Prevent or work to reduce common risk and environmental factors that contribute to:

    • decline in physical functional

    • impaired quality of life

    • social isolation

    • excess disability in older adults

15. Assist the patient to compensate for age-related functional changes according to chronological age groups

16. Refer and/or manage common signs, symptoms and syndromes (with consideration of setting, environment, population, comorbidities, and multiple contributing factors), with specific attention to:

    • immobility, risk of falls, gait disturbance

    • incontinence

    • cognitive impairment (depression, delirium, dementia)

- nutritional compromise
- substance use/abuse
- abuse or neglect (verbal, physical, and sexual)
- suicide or homicide ideations

17. Maintain or maximize muscle function and mobility, continence, mood, memory and orientation, nutrition, and hydration

18. Use an ethical framework to address individual and family concerns about caregiving, management of pain, and end-of-life issues

19. Strive for restraint-free care, minimizing the use of physical and chemical restraints, and develop the most independent and protective setting possible

20. Account for cognitive, sensory, and perceptual problems, with special attention to temperature sensation, hearing, and vision when caring for older adults

21. Recognize the heightened need for coordination of care with other health care providers and community resources, with special attention to the frail older adult and those with markedly advanced age

22. Develop caring relationships with patients, families, and other caregivers to address sensitive issues, such as driving, independent living, potential for abuse, end-of-life issues, advanced directives, and finances

23. Review treatment options and facilitate decision-making with the patient, family, and other caregivers or the patient's health care proxy

24. Consider age-related changes when executing teaching-coaching with regards to sensory and perceptual limitations, cognitive limitations, and memory changes

25. Utilize adult learning principles in patient, family, and caregiver education, such as timing of teaching, longer time to learn and respond, and need for individualized instruction, integration of information, and use of multiple strategies of communication

26. Educate older adults, families, and caregivers about normal vs. abnormal events, physiological changes with aging, and myths of aging

27. Educate older adults, family, and caregivers about the need for preventive health care and end-of-life choices

28. Disseminate knowledge of skills required to care for older adults to other health care workers and caregivers through peer education, staff development, and preceptor experiences

29. Advocate within the health care system and policy arenas for the health needs of older adults, especially the frail and markedly advanced older adult

30. Articulate and promote to other health care providers and the public, the role within the health care team of either the NP or CNS, and its significance in improving outcomes of care for older adults

31. Create and enhance positive, health-promoting environments that maintain a climate of dignity and privacy for older adults

32. Understand payment and reimbursement systems and financial resources across the continuum of care

33. Promote continuity of care and manage transitions across the continuum of care

34. Communicate to other members of the interdisciplinary care team special needs of the older adult to improve outcomes of care

35. Collaborate with the interdisciplinary geriatric and geropsychiatric care team to improve outcomes of care

36. Participate in the design and implementation of evidence-based protocols and processes of care to reduce adverse events common to older adults, such as infections, falls, and polypharmacy

37. Address the impact of ageism, sexism, and cultural biases on health care policies and systems

38. Use public and private databases to incorporate evidence-based practices into the care of older adults

39. Apply evidence-based practice using quality improvement methodologies in providing quality care to older adults

40. Use available technology to enhance safety and monitor the health status and outcomes of older adults

41. Facilitate access to hospice and palliative care to maximize a peaceful, pain-free, and compassionate death for patients with any end-stage disease, including dementia

42. Assesses intergenerational differences in family members' beliefs that influence care, e.g., end-of-life care

43. Recognize the potential for cultural and ethnic differences between patients and multiple caregivers to impact outcomes of care

44. Assess patients' and caregivers' cultural and spiritual priorities as part of a holistic assessment

45. Adapt age-specific assessment methods or tools to a culturally diverse population

46. Educate professional and lay caregivers to provide culturally competent care to older adults

47. Incorporate culturally and spiritually appropriate resources into the planning and delivery of health care

Source: American Association of Colleges (AACN). (2004). *Nurse practitioner and clinical nurse specialist competencies for older adult care*. Washington, DC: AACN, pp. 6–9.

AACN/JAHF Competencies Integrated Within the NONPF 2002 Domains of Nurse Practitioner Practice

Domain	Competencies
I. Health Promotion, Health Protection, Disease Prevention, and Treatment	
A. Assessment of Health Status	1. Differentiate normal aging from illness and disease processes.
	2. Use standardized assessment instruments appropriate to older adults if available, or a standardized assessment process to assess social support and health status, such as function; cognition; mobility; pain; skin integrity; quality of life; nutrition; neglect and abuse.
	3. Assess for syndromes, constellations of symptoms that may be manifestations of other health problems, common to older adults, e.g., incontinence, falling, delirium, dementia, and depression.
	4. Assess health status and identify risk factors in older adults.
	5. Assess the ability of the individual and family to manage developmental (life stage) transitions, resilience, and coping strategies.
	6. Assess older adult's, family's, and caregiver's ability to execute plans of care.

(Continued)

Domain	Competencies
	7. Conduct a pharmacological assessment of the older adult, including polypharmacy, drug interactions, over-the-counter and herbal product use, and ability to obtain, purchase medications, and safely and correctly self-administer medications.
	8. Assess for pain in the older adult, including the cognitively impaired, and develop a plan of care to manage.
B. Diagnosis of Health Status	9. Identify both typical and atypical manifestations of chronic and acute illnesses and diseases common to older adults.
	10. Recognize the presence of co-morbidities and iatrogenesis in the frail older adult.
	11. Identify signs and symptoms indicative of change in mental status, e.g., agitation, anxiety, depression, substance use, delirium, and dementia.
	12. Interpret results of appropriate laboratory and diagnostic tests, differentiating values for older adults.
C. Plan of Care and Implementation of Treatment	13. Promote and recommend immunizations and appropriate health screenings.
	14. Prevent or work to reduce common risk and environmental factors that contribute to: • decline in physical function • impaired quality of life • social isolation • excess disability in older adults
	15. Assist the patient to compensate for age-related functional changes according to chronological age groups.
	16. Refer and/or manage common signs, symptoms, and syndromes (with consideration of setting, environment, population, co-morbidities, and multiple contributing factors), with specific attention to: • immobility, risk of falls, gait disturbance • incontinence • cognitive impairment (depression, delirium, dementia) • nutritional compromise • substance use/abuse • abuse or neglect (verbal, physical, and sexual) • suicide or homicide ideations

Domain	Competencies
	17. Maintain or maximize muscle function and mobility, continence, mood, memory and orientation, nutrition, and hydration.
	18. Use an ethical framework to address individual and family concerns about caregiving, management of pain, and end-of-life issues.
	19. Strive for restraint-free care, minimizing the use of physical and chemical restraints, and develop the most independent and protective setting possible.
II. The Nurse Practitioner– Patient Relationship	20. Account for cognitive, sensory, and perceptual problems with special attention to temperature sensation, hearing and vision when caring for older adults.
	21. Recognize the heightened need for coordination of care with other health care providers and community resources with special attention to the frail older adult and those with markedly advanced age.
	22. Develop caring relationships with patients, families, and other caregivers to address sensitive issues, such as driving, independent living, potential for abuse, end-of-life issues, advanced directives, and finances.
	23. Review treatment options and facilitate decision-making with the patient, family, and other caregivers or the patient's health care proxy.
III. The Teaching– Coaching Function	24. Consider age-related changes when executing teaching-coaching with regard to sensory and perceptual limitations, cognitive limitations, and memory changes
	25. Utilize adult learning principles in patient, family, and caregiver education, such as timing of teaching, longer time to learn and respond, and need for individualized instruction, integration of information, and use of multiple strategies of communication.
	26. Educate older adults, family, and caregivers about normal vs. abnormal events, physiological changes with aging, and myths of aging.
	27. Educate older adults, families, and caregivers about the need for preventive health care and end-of-life choices.
	28. Disseminate knowledge of skills required to care for older adults to other health care workers and caregivers through peer education, staff development, and preceptor experiences.

(Continued)

Domain	Competencies
IV. Professional Role	29. Advocate within the health care system and policy arenas for the health needs of older adults, especially the frail and markedly advanced older adult.
	30. Articulate and promote to other health care providers and the public, the role within the health care team, of either the NP or CNS, and its significance in improving outcomes of care for older adults.
	31. Create and enhance positive, health-promoting environments that maintain a climate of dignity and privacy for older adults.
V. Managing and Negotiating Health Care Delivery Systems	32. Understand payment and reimbursement systems and financial resources across the continuum of care.
	33. Promote continuity of care and manage transitions across the continuum of care.
	34. Communicate to other members of the interdisciplinary care team special needs of the older adult to improve outcomes of care.
	35. Collaborate with the interdisciplinary geriatric and geropsychiatric care team to improve outcomes of care.
	36. Participate in the design and implementation of evidence-based protocols and processes of care to reduce adverse events common to older adults, such as infections, falls, polypharmacy.
VI. Monitoring and Ensuring the Quality of Health Care Practice	37. Address the impact of ageism, sexism, and cultural biases on health care policies and systems.
	38. Use public and private databases to incorporate evidence-based practices into the care of older adults.
	39. Apply evidence-based practice using quality improvement methodologies in providing quality care to older adults.
	40. Use available technology to enhance safety and monitor the health status and outcomes of older adults.
	41. Facilitate access to hospice and palliative care to maximize a peaceful, pain-free, and compassionate death for patients with any end-stage disease, including dementia.

Domain	Competencies
VII. Cultural and Spiritual Competence	42. Assess intergenerational differences in family members' beliefs that influence care, e.g., end-of-life care.
	43. Recognize the potential for cultural and ethnic differences between patients and multiple caregivers to impact outcomes of care.
	44. Assess patients' and caregivers' cultural and spiritual priorities as part of a holistic assessment.
	45. Adapt age-specific assessment methods or tools to a culturally diverse population.
	46. Educate professional and lay caregivers to provide culturally competent care to older adults.
	47. Incorporate culturally and spiritually appropriate resources into the planning and delivery of health care.

Source: American Association of Colleges (AACN). (2004). *Nurse practitioner and clinical nurse specialist competencies for older adult care.* Washington, DC: AACN, pp. 11–15.

AACN/JAHF Competencies Integrated Within the NACNS 2004 Clinical Nurse Specialist Spheres of Influence

Sphere of Influence	Competencies
I. Patient/Client	
A. Assessment B. Diagnosis, Planning, and Interventions C. Evaluation	1. Differentiate normal aging from illness and disease processes. 2. Use standardized assessment instruments appropriate to older adults if available, or a standardized assessment process to assess social support and health status, such as function; cognition; mobility; pain; skin integrity; quality of life; nutrition; neglect and abuse. 3. Assess for syndromes, constellations of symptoms that may be manifestations of other health problems common to older adults, e.g., incontinence, falling, delirium, dementia, and depression. 4. Assess health status and identify risk factors in older adults. 5. Assess the ability of the individual and family to manage developmental (life stage) transitions, resilience, and coping strategies. 6. Assess older adult's, family's, and caregiver's ability to execute plans of care. 7. Conduct a pharmacological assessment of the older adult, including polypharmacy, drug interactions, over-the-counter and herbal product use, and ability to obtain, purchase medications, and safely and correctly self-administer medications. 8. Assess for pain in the older adult, including the cognitively impaired, and develop a plan of care to manage.

(Continued)

Sphere of Influence	Competencies

9. Identify both typical and atypical manifestations of chronic and acute illnesses and diseases common to older adults.

10. Recognize the presence of co-morbidities and iatrogenesis in the frail older adult.

11. Identify signs and symptoms indicative of change in mental status, e.g., agitation, anxiety, depression, substance use, delirium, and dementia.

12. Interpret results of appropriate laboratory and diagnostic tests, differentiating values for older adults.

13. Promote and recommend immunizations and appropriate health screenings.

14. Prevent or work to reduce common risk and environmental factors that contribute to:
    - decline in physical function
    - impaired quality of life
    - social isolation
    - excess disability in older adults

15. Assist the patient to compensate for age-related functional changes according to chronological age groups.

16. Refer and/or manage common signs, symptoms, and syndromes (with consideration of setting, environment, population, co-morbidities, and multiple contributing factors), with specific attention to:
    - immobility, risk of falls, gait disturbance
    - incontinence
    - cognitive impairment (depression, delirium, dementia)
    - nutritional compromise
    - substance use/abuse
    - abuse or neglect (verbal, physical, and sexual)
    - suicide or homicide ideations

17. Maintain or maximize muscle function and mobility, continence, mood, memory and orientation, nutrition, and hydration.

18. Use an ethical framework to address individual and family concerns about caregiving, management of pain, and end-of-life issues.

19. Strive for restraint-free care, minimizing the use of physical and chemical restraints, and develop the most independent and protective setting possible.

Sphere of Influence	Competencies
	20. Account for cognitive, sensory, and perceptual problems with special attention to temperature sensation, hearing, and vision when caring for older adults.
	21. Recognize the heightened need for coordination of care with other health care providers and community resources, with special attention to the frail older adult and those with markedly advanced age.
	22. Develop caring relationships with patients, families, and other caregivers to address sensitive issues, such as driving, independent living, potential for abuse, end-of-life issues, advanced directives, and finances.
	23. Review treatment options and facilitate decision-making with the patient, family, and other caregivers or the patient's health care proxy.
	24. Consider age-related changes when executing teaching-coaching with regard to sensory and perceptual limitations, cognitive limitations, and memory changes.
	25. Utilize adult learning principles in patient, family, and caregiver education, such as timing of teaching, longer time to learn and respond, and need for individualized instruction, integration of information, and use of multiple strategies of communication.
	26. Educate older adults, family, and caregivers about normal vs. abnormal events, physiological changes with aging, and myths of aging.
	27. Educate older adults, families, and caregivers about the need for preventive health care and end-of-life choices.
	32. Understand payment and reimbursement systems and financial resources across the continuum of care.
	40. Use available technology to enhance safety and monitor the health status and outcomes of older adults.
	41. Facilitate access to hospice and palliative care to maximize a peaceful, pain-free, and compassionate death for patients with any end-stage disease, including dementia.
	42. Assess intergenerational differences in family members' beliefs that influence care, e.g., end-of-life care.
	43. Recognize the potential for cultural and ethnic differences between patients and multiple caregivers to impact outcomes of care.

(Continued)

Sphere of Influence	Competencies

	44. Assess patients' and caregivers' cultural and spiritual priorities as part of a holistic assessment.
	45. Adapt age-specific assessment methods or tools to a culturally diverse population.
	Competencies 1–27, 32, 40–45.

II. Nurses and
Nursing Practice

A. Assessment — Competencies 1–12.

B. Diagnosis,
Planning, and
Intervention

C. Evaluation

Competencies 13–27, 32, 40–46, as well as

28. Disseminate knowledge of skills required to care for older adults to other health care workers and caregivers through peer education, staff development, and preceptor experiences.

29. Advocate within the health care system and policy arenas for the health needs of older adults, especially the frail and markedly advanced older adult.

30. Articulate and promote to other health care providers and the public, the role within the health care team, of either the NP or CNS, and its significance in improving outcomes of care for older adults.

31. Create and enhance positive, health-promoting environments that maintain a climate of dignity and privacy for older adults.

33. Promote continuity of care and manage transitions across the continuum of care.

34. Communicate to other members of the interdisciplinary care team special needs of the older adult to improve outcomes of care.

35. Collaborate with the interdisciplinary geriatric and geropsychiatric care team to improve outcomes of care.

36. Participate in the design and implementation of evidence-based protocols and processes of care to reduce adverse events common to older adults, such as infections, falls, polypharmacy.

37. Address the impact of ageism, sexism, and cultural biases on health care policies and systems.

38. Use public and private databases to incorporate evidence-based practices into the care of older adults.

Sphere of Influence	Competencies
	39. Apply evidence-based practice using quality improvement methodologies in providing quality care to older adults.
	46. Educate professional and lay caregivers to provide culturally competent care to older adults.
	47. Incorporate culturally and spiritually appropriate resources into the planning and delivery of health care.

III. Organization/ System
  A. Assessment
  B. Diagnosis, Planning and Intervention
  C. Evaluation
	Competencies 1–47
	CNS competencies for care of older adults in the organization/system sphere include: Competencies 18, 19, 21–22, 27–41, 43, 47

Source: American Association of Colleges (AACN). (2004). *Nurse practitioner and clinical nurse specialist competencies for older adult care.* Washington, DC: AACN, pp. 16–22.

Integration of Gerontological Content Worksheet

Course	Content	Competencies	Learning Strategies	Evaluation Methods
Research				
Theory				
Health Policy				
Professional Roles				
Pathophysiology				

Course	Content	Competencies	Learning Strategies	Evaluation Methods
Pharmacology				
Physical/Health Assessment				
Health Promotion and Prevention Focus				
Diagnosis and Management Courses				
Independent Study in Geriatrics				

Source: © 2009 Laurie Kennedy-Malone, PhD, GNP-BC, FAANP, FAGHE, Carolyn Auerhahn, EdD, ANP, GNP-BC, FAANP, Evelyn Groenke Duffy, DNP, G/ANP-BC, FAANP

Index